ØYVIND TORP

GEIR STIAN ULSTEIN

Self-Defence Against Cancer

Ten counter-moves you can use

First published in the Norwegian language as *Selvforsvar mot kreft* by
Øyvind Torp & Geir Stian Ulstein
Spartacus forlag, Oslo, Norway, 2020

First published in English 2020
Copyright © 2020 Øyvind Torp & Geir Stian Ulstein
English translation Frank Stewart

Coverdesign: Kjetil Waren Johnsen / Wisuell Design
Authorportrait: Tor Simen Ulstein
Bookdesign: Torp-Land-Ulstein Design

Disclaimer: The methods and measures in this book are meant as compliments to - not as replacements for- standard medical treatment. The authors and publisher of this book are not liable for any personal   injury or damage that may arise through improper application and a failure of the individual to seek correct medical advice with any of the treatments outlined in this book.

Contents

DR ØYVIND TORP

FOREWORD

When I was diagnosed with cancer in June 2016, the news shook my world to its foundations. My solid confidence in the future was suddenly replaced by an unstable tower of harsh, unanswerable questions.

Why me? What have I done wrong? How will this end?

Fortunately, another important question also arose. What can I do to improve my prognosis?

I would obviously have to follow the doctors' advice and accept the recommended treatment and follow-up. We discussed the various options of surgery, chemotherapy and radiation.

I was grateful that these treatment programmes were available, but how could I contribute in the intervals between the important medical interventions?

I was naturally keen to play an active part in the struggle for my life, but the cancer specialists shook their heads: 'So long as you don't smoke, we have nothing else to recommend.'

I felt powerless.

The questions continued. Why should an otherwise fit 39-year old man get cancer? Was it sheer bad luck?

As a doctor I had a basic knowledge of cancer. I knew that over 90 per cent of cases of cancer were caused by environmental factors such as tobacco smoking, obesity, excessive alcohol intake, radiation, unhealthy diet and lack of physical activity. However, I didn't really know what a diagnosis of cancer meant. I would soon find out. Getting cancer is bad luck, but had I done something to open the door to bad luck?

I pondered what might have led to the disease in my case. Could it be diet? I didn't smoke. I did not drink very much alcohol, and was not overweight. I didn't need to know the answer to punish myself, but I needed to know whether stopping anything that could have increased my risk of cancer might help. I could not accept the idea that there was no point in doing anything to help myself. My thoughts went further. Why should the measures that were recommended for the prevention of cancer not be just as important at the onset of the disease?

I started reading about the topic. In the literature I found masses of information about measures that could slow down and counteract the disease in combination with surgery, chemotherapy or radiation. I found new possibilities to improve my chances. In the midst of fear, catastrophising and despair, I needed to absorb myself in a project. I needed to take an active part in the fight for my own life. I developed strategies that dissipated my pervasive negative thoughts in the waiting times between series of investigations and operations. I was able to focus more on how I could improve my own prospects in face of the apparently bleak outlook. I felt better and better, both physically and emotionally.

The act of taking an active part and contributing positively to my own treatment, taking responsibility for my own fate, gave me a sense of relief, purpose and hope.

That is also the basic idea behind this book.

I hope that you will be inspired to start your own project, enabling you to take meaningful steps on the way towards better health.

The book is divided into three main parts. The first part describes the nature and causes of cancer.

In the second part, I point out that cancer also has weak points that you can take advantage of.

The third and final part offers practical advice on how you can best carry out a counter-attack on cancer and suggests ten steps in increasing order of difficulty. You may not necessarily have motivation or energy to follow all my advice, but re-

member that each individual measure is effective.
You can do it!

Øyvind Torp
1,000 days after cancer diagnosis.

THE DREAM OF RUNNING

T he wheels on the drip-stand rattle as I make my way down the corridor towards the cafeteria in the National Hospital. Hanging on the stand is a plastic bag containing morphine solution. I only have to press a button on the pump to send a dose of the painkiller down the tube and into my spinal canal. The nerves are anaesthetised. I need a dose of morphine to accomplish my expedition from the ward to the coffee machine.

This is my target for the evening.

The National Hospital has a distinctive air of calm at eventide. High ceilings absorb the noise. From the hospital entrance, the main corridor runs like a street the whole length of the building. It's a village street with paving slabs and street lamps, and 'houses' standing close together with varying pillars and facades. Here and there are terraces, though you never see anyone using them. In the street there are green trees and plants, steps to sit on and piazzas in which to congregate, each with its characteristic sculptures. It could almost be a pleasant street in a quiet Italian village. But it is a street for people whose lives are at risk.

I remember when King Harald proudly and officially opened the National Hospital on 22nd September 2000. As a very fresh medical student, I was in the male choir providing entertainment on this great day. In my years as a student, I spent many hours roaming these corridors to visit patients in various wards. I had no thought of soon being a patient here myself.

My current companion on the road is the drip-stand. I pull it along, being careful not to entangle the plastic tubing in the small wheels. Ahead looms a journey of a hundred metres.

Fourteen days earlier – two days before the operation – I completed a triathlon. I had felt in top form. I remember how I could press on though the water before jumping up onto the bike and pressing on again. I can see myself on the bicycle pedalling rapidly to dance up the steep slopes and then launch fearlessly into an increasingly rapid descent. I remember the taste of blood in my mouth during the running phase, I remember managing to regulate my metabolism and my activity to avoid developing lactic acidosis. I remember crossing the finishing line. And then the wonderful feeling of achievement, fatigue and satisfaction. That was fourteen days ago.

That was a different life.

Right now, this short walk in the National Hospital seems humanly impossible.

I eventually reach the kiosk. A hundred metres covered. It seems like a greater achievement than the triathlon, but I am too worn out to rejoice.

I realise that the way back to my former fit and healthy body is a long road. But it could have been worse. There may be a little, narrow bridge, a glimmer of hope, that can take me back there. I need a dream to follow, something to work on, something to lift me out of this valley of gloom.

That night, I dreamed of running the Berlin marathon.

DIAGNOSIS: BECOMING A PATIENT

I t was early summer 2016. My consulting room was rather too warm, and I was sweating a little in my suit. I couldn't gather my thoughts. It was as if I had been hit in the stomach by a canon-ball.

Two patients were sitting waiting in the corridor. I ought to have taken them in a long time ago, but I was completely out of action.

My hands moved rather shakily over the keyboard. Black letters glared at me from the screen. I looked at the text again. Could the news be different this time? No, the radiologist's report left no doubt.

I had opened my in-box and been confronted by the image and report of my own MRI scan. I had opened the report without hesitation, not expecting to be faced with catastrophe.

'Tumours in the pancreas. Widespread enlarged lymph nodes in the abdomen. Tumour in a rib.'

I felt queasy. I ought to have gone straight home, but it would have been difficult to cancel the patients who were waiting. The very last one was suffering from depression. I called her in. It was a relief to concentrate on the patient and feel that I was helping her.

To a young medical student, disease was of academic interest. It was theory, it was a subject of study, it didn't apply to me personally. But I was moved by the plight of many patients, and cancer patients made a particularly strong impression on a young student. It was such a sad fate which seemed to me at that time to be a death-sentence, though we also saw that treatment could be effective. I really think that I found this disease so frightening as a student that I later did my best to ignore the symptoms that came over me in the course of several years.

You would think that a doctor would be particularly well prepared when struck by disease, but the truth is that over the years I distanced myself from any thought of being ill myself. When one lives with and experiences so much disease and so many sad outcomes, it is perhaps natural to protect oneself by suppressing such thoughts. It is said that some doctors have been so good at suppressing their own symptoms that when they are diagnosed with serious disease, it has progressed so far that they are beyond saving. Was I one of those?

And why do so many people get cancer?

PART 1:
WHAT IS CANCER?

CANCER - AN EPIDEMIC?

I n the USA, cancer is now almost the most frequent cause of death. One in two men and one in three women in the USA can expect to be struck by cancer at some time in their life. Cancer has become more prevalent* in all western countries since 1940 and increasingly so since 1973, especially among younger members of the populations. In Norway, for example, 36 per cent of men and 30 per cent of women will probably have been affected by cancer by the time they have reached the age of 75.1

The incidence** of cancer among people in the USA under the age of 45 has been increasing each year by 1.6 per cent among women and 1.8 per cent among men. Between 1970 and 1999 the combined incidence of cancer increased by 1.0 per cent among children and 1.5 per cent among young people.[2] In France, the total incidence of all cancers increased by 60 per cent from 1977 to 2000.[3]

An explanation that is frequently offered is that the population is becoming older and therefore more at risk of cancer. However, children and young people are among the sections of the population where the incidence of cancer has risen most since the 1970s. So there is an increase in *all* age-groups. Nor can the increase be explained by better diagnosis, for the increase is at least as high among types of cancer for which there are no screening programmes (lung, brain, testicle, pancreas, lymphatic system) as it is among the types we have become good at diagnosing early.

What lies behind this alarming increase?

* Prevalence: the number of cases in a particular population at a particular time (e.g. x cases per y people on d date) * Incidence: the number of new cases in a particular population within a particular time (e.g. x new cases per y people per year)

WHY ME?

Bent over the news on the computer screen, I started wondering about cancer from a biological point of view. As a family doctor, this was not my special field. We are generalists, taking an overview of most symptoms and illnesses. One of our roles is to suspect or detect cancer so that treatment can be started early enough. When necessary we can give further advice or confer with the oncologists. Now, facing the disease myself, I felt a need to know all the details.

It is easy to be confused by the body's incredibly complicated and finely tuned mechanisms. Despite the multiplicity of functions that cells and organs have to perform and the enormous complexity of the systems by which they work, the body usually functions without problems. The cells divide, produce proteins, communicate with each other and when necessary, sacrifice themselves in the best interests of the organism as a whole. However, faults do regularly crop up that could lead to serious consequences. The reason for this is not clear, but the result is what we call cancer.

Cancer is not a distinct disease, but a group of diseases whose common feature is that the body has lost control over parts of the cell division. Cell division is happening all the time. Most cells are replaced regularly. The process of cell division is controlled by genes. When a gene governing cell division undergoes changes – 'mutations' – cell division can run out of control. A simple over-proliferation of cells can lead to benign swellings such as warts and polyps. 'Benign' simply means that the tumour doesn't spread further. But during such uncontrolled cell growth, some cells can undergo changes that lead them to spread wider, becoming 'malignant.' That is a dramatic situation for the body to deal with.

Cancer cells break loose and are carried in the lymphatic circulation or through the bloodstream to other parts of the body. The tumour can also invade neighbouring tissues directly. In these ways, the cancer cells embed themselves in healthy tissue where they multiply further to produce new tumours, known as 'metastases.'

It usually takes many years for a malignant tumour to become big enough to cause symptoms. By the time a cancerous tumour has spread, it is usually incurable. It is difficult to eradicate and is frequently though not invariably fatal. Treatment can prolong life and improve quality of life.

I felt crushed as I sat in my office with the computer screen shimmering before my eyes. What could I do about this impossible disease? I was entering unknown territory.

The next few weeks were unreal. I wakened up every day with a painful feeling in my stomach. Had it just been a nightmare? Then every morning the truth struck me like lightning. A new chapter had begun in my life, made up of investigations, catastrophic fears and meetings with more and more doctors. I found being at the other side of the desk a very unfamiliar role.

When I was admitted to the National Hospital, I felt reluctant to take off my 'civilian' clothes, put on the hospital 'uniform' and lie down on a hospital bed. I felt fit. The change of role was so strange for me that later, during my convalescence, I took every opportunity to change back into my own clothes and roam the corridors as I had done of old, before I was condemned to act as a patient. The change between 'health' and 'sickness' had come far too suddenly. My whole identity was in question. I had lost myself; I was no longer strong and healthy. I didn't even feel like a doctor any more; I was signed off sick; I had become a patient. Losing control over my own life was frightening.

I was grieving over a life that would be foreshortened, years that I would not experience, moments I would not be able to share with my nearest and dearest. I felt pained that I could not be a father, not be a husband. Not be. Who would take my place?

Fortunately there were counterweights to these depressing thoughts. The oncologists were skilled professionals who were able to deal with my questions and redirect my thoughts from spinning off too far in unhelpful directions. I was treated well, by able professionals with both empathy and knowledge.

I had also drawn the winning ticket in another area; I experienced warm and moving support from family and friends. Hanne, my wife for ten years, was by my side all the time. It was good to be a twosome when hard news had to be absorbed and difficult questions faced. She had to drive the car when the reports had been heavy to bear and I couldn't concentrate on the traffic. What's more, she is a psychiatrist. She taught me the benefit of sorting out my thoughts and not necessarily trusting every idea that passed through my head.

Thoughts are only thoughts.

If I thought that I had incurable cancer, that was not necessarily true. There might be an effective treatment. Anyway, I could think about living and enjoying life for a good while yet.

Nobody can choose how long they have left, but I could choose to believe that there were possibilities of treatment and improvement.

'Is there another way of looking at this?' Hanne often asked. 'Is it really so bad, or is that just how you have interpreted it?'

She often uses such cognitive techniques in her practice as a psychiatrist. Now I was in a sense her patient.

I underwent an operation in June 2016 and tried to build myself up physically for the next one in August. I knew this one would be harder.

At the same time, I had started researching the subject in more depth. I needed to read everything I could find about cancer. I was looking for the disease's weak points. If I found any, I would make use of them.

My urge to fight grew as I found more and more information about the disease's vulnerabilities. The faint hope within me flared up. There were so many stories out there about people who had improved their own prognosis by adding their own efforts to the treatment that was offered to them.

I hadn't known about this before. And I found many such trails to follow.

Was it possible to fight back?

I never thought for a moment of rejecting the oncologists' advice about treatment. My 'project' would be a supplement to the usual treatment, not an alternative.

I searched the literature further. I needed to know more about the disease to establish why I had been afflicted. Reading about this now was however much more frightening than reading about it as a student. It now affected me directly. I noted with horror what the cancer cells do to the body. They were described as outlaws ransacking their surroundings for nourishment and ignoring the rules that healthy cells have to obey. Among other things, cancer cells refuse to die after a certain number of cell divisions. They circumvent the body's defence mechanisms when adjacent healthy cells ask them to stop dividing. They also contaminate the surrounding tissue with their secretions. This leads to inflammation that stimulate even more invasive growth of the tumour. The cancer cells commandeer the blood supply and become self-sustaining so that they can grow faster. They compel the blood vessels to divide and grow to supply the tumour with oxygen and nutrients.

That is cancer's strength. Only slowly and with good help from international research literature did I realise that there were also weaknesses that could be put to use.

I always came back to the nagging question: *Why me?* Was it because of a secret inheritance of insidious, unknown genes?

I remember asking a lecturer, 'Is this disease inherited?' 'Everything is inherited,' he replied. 'We can't escape our genetic inheritance,' I thought sadly.

But now I had begun to explore new, exciting research that is changing views of our genetic fate. Perhaps genes are not so inevitably determinant of fate after all. A harmful gene can be switched off and become inactive with favourable effect, and on the other hand a beneficial gene can be activated.

In this way, environmental influences can lead to changes. The emotional stress of a traumatic childhood, for example, can have epigenetic effects that lead to depression later in life.[4] Living in a contaminated environment or eating food that slowly poisons the body can have similar effects. Epigenetic changes such as this are probably the reason why among identical twins with the same genetic predisposition to schizophrenia, the disease affects both twins in less than 50 per cent of cases.

Were there any factors predisposing to cancer in my case, or had I just been unlucky? I needed to find out, not to rebuke myself for something I could have done otherwise but to consider whether the factors that had led to my cancer could be tackled in order to improve my prognosis. That would be useful.

It is quite clear to me that nobody is guilty for getting cancer. We all know somebody who has smoked like a chimney for years but nevertheless lives long over the expected age. I have known super-fit people who have died all too soon. I have had patients who got lung cancer without ever having used tobacco. Such extremely bad luck seems unfair.

I wanted to know more about the different factors that predispose to cancer. These showed up clearly in international research reports.[5]

The most prominent factor was smoking, an important cause of about 35 per cent of cases. Second was diet, which contributed to 30 per cent of cases. Exposure to harmful substances at work was responsible for 15 to 20 per cent. These included asbestos, radiation and various gases and other chemicals. Infections such as Helicobacter Pylori, Hepatitis B and C, Human Papilloma Virus (HPV) and Epstein Barr Virus accounted for 10 per cent.

From this, I calculated that only 5 to 10 per cent of the total risk of cancer can be attributed to heredity (genes), bad luck and chance.

This was a revelation to me. Even though it was bad luck for me to get cancer as an individual, it is not just bad luck on a population level. Perhaps only 5 or 10 per cent of cases of cancer are purely genetically determined. So environmental factors are important in 90 to 95 per cent of cases.

Just think if we could live in a world that didn't trigger the risk of cancer!
If these figures are correct, we as a society could prevent nine out of ten cases of cancer if we managed to:
Avoid tobacco;
Avoid exposure to harmful chemicals, radiation and so on at work;
Vaccinate ourselves against cancer-inducing viruses such as hepatitis C and Human Papilloma Virus;
Treat the harmful stomach bacterium Helicobacter Pylori if we are infected;
Eat an optimal diet.

It was too late for me now, but could I have done anything different earlier?

I couldn't have done very much about pollution in the air and in food. I had avoided smoking and had taken alcohol only moderately, but I had got cancer nevertheless. Nor could I have done anything about my genes. So there remained only one risk factor that I could tackle.

Even though I was a qualified doctor, I didn't know that I perhaps should have thought more about my diet. I thought it had been quite healthy. I had thought of my diet with regard to weight and training. I hadn't considered invisible long-term effects – for we are not yet taught anything about that.

There didn't appear to be a problem with my diet at first glance, but on closer investigation it became apparent. The more I read, the more I saw that a 'normal Norwegian diet' is not necessarily healthy. Many people are at risk from far too great quantities of carbohydrate in their diet. But here too there are differences. Some people appear to cope well with living on a carbohydrate-based diet, whereas others tolerate it badly, develop lifestyle diseases such as obesity and diabetes and also become at risk of cancer.

Despite the advice from health authorities that wholemeal bread, wholemeal pasta, potatoes, milk and lots of fruit are all healthy, one can also have *too much* of them. Carbohydrates are broken down to sugar in the small bowel. In addition, we are eating rather large quantities of sugar. Norwegians eat an average of 27 kg. of sugar per person each year,[6] most Western Europeans between about 30 and 36 kg. and Americans about 46 kg. On top of the masses of other carbohydrates, this can add up to a remarkably and unnaturally high total.

After the concern about dietary fats arose in the mid 1980s, we have obediently followed the advice to reduce fatty foods. These have been replaced by carbohydrates. The total of all carbohydrates in the diet can be really high, when one takes into account both the 'healthy' unrefined varieties and the refined, sweet varieties such as cakes, biscuits, juice, sweets, snacks and sugar. These all end up as glucose sugar when they are broken down in the small bowel. Our sugar intake is higher than we realise – certainly higher than I realised.

Not everybody can tolerate such a high load of sugar, and it may be one of the main reasons for the increase in overweight and diabetes we have seen in recent years since we were advised to reduce our consumption of fats and have replaced these with carbohydrates. The incidence of cancer has risen correspondingly, showing that overweight and diabetes are closely related to cancer risk.[7]

Had my own diet perhaps sometimes have been a little less healthy than average? I am very fond of sweet things, especially cakes. On reflection, I realise that I might have eaten more than just a few sweet things each day.

I began to calculate. A litre of juice generally contains 100 g. of sugar, equivalent to 50 sugar cubes, even though the carton is labelled 'no added sugar.'[8]

I made similar discoveries time after time when I began reading the lists of contents. Jam 'with no added sugar' was nevertheless full of it. The yoghurt I thought was healthy contributed numerous 'sugar cubes' to my intake. And then there were pasta, potatoes, bread and rice all being rapidly converted into glucose as soon as they reached the small bowel. I had been eating large amounts of sugar without realising it. I hadn't been very good at eating fish either, and I was not very taken with vegetables.

My self-examination had begun. I had been unlucky to get cancer, but I would use the knowledge of its causes sensibly.

How common is cancer?

In 2018, an estimated 1,735,350 new cases of cancer will be diagnosed in the United States and 609,640 people will die from the disease.

The most common cancers (listed in descending order according to estimated new cases in 2018) are breast cancer, lung and bronchus cancer, prostate cancer, colon and rectum cancer, melanoma of the skin, bladder cancer, non-Hodgkin lymphoma, kidney and renal pelvis cancer, endometrial cancer, leukemia, pancreatic cancer, thyroid cancer, and liver cancer.

The number of new cases of cancer (cancer incidence) is 439.2 per 100,000 men and women per year (based on 2011–2015 cases).

The number of cancer deaths (cancer mortality) is 163.5 per 100,000 men and women per year (based on 2011–2015 deaths).

Cancer mortality is higher among men than women (196.8 per 100,000 men and 139.6 per 100,000 women). When comparing groups based on race/ethnicity and sex, cancer mortality is highest in African American men (239.9 per 100,000) and lowest in Asian/Pacific Islander women (88.3 per 100,000).

In 2016, there were an estimated 15.5 million cancer survivors in the United States. The number of cancer survivors is expected to increase to 20.3 million by 2026.

Approximately 38.4% of men and women will be diagnosed with cancer at some point during their lifetimes (based on 2013–2015 data).

In 2017, an estimated 15,270 children and adolescents ages 0 to 19 were diagnosed with cancer and 1,790 died of the disease.

Estimated national expenditures for cancer care in the United States in 2017 were $147.3 billion. In future years, costs are likely to increase as the population ages and cancer prevalence increases. Costs are also likely to increase as new, and often more expensive, treatments are adopted as standards of care.

In Norway in 2016, 32,827 people were diagnosed with cancer. Of these, 15,064 were women and 17,763 were men. In 2015 there were 262,884 people in Norway living with cancer.[9]

WHY ISN'T CANCER CURED?

O n 23rd December 1971, American President Richard Nixon declared 'war against cancer.' Scientists and the general population were optimistic following enormous advances in technology and medicine during the previous decades. Many people imagined that the cancer puzzle would at last be solved.

Enormous sums are now being devoted to research. However, even though we have made big advances in understanding cancer at a genetic and molecular level, few advances have been made towards finding a cure – with the exception of some types of leukaemia and some types of cancer where immunotherapy has proved itself effective (at least temporarily) in some patients. Sadly, we appear to be as far from finding a cure now as we were when Nixon declared war on the disease. After half a century and enormous expenditure we are still on the defensive.

HOW DOES
CANCER START?

Cancer was now my new personal enemy. I began to wonder what it really was, from a biological point of view. I hoped that if I understood my enemy thoroughly, I could find his weak points.

The literature records several theories of why cancer starts. For a long time, the most widely accepted theory has been somatic mutation. Genetic mutations occur frequently in the body under normal conditions, but most of the 'mistakes' that happen will be detected and repaired by the body's defence mechanisms. Occasionally a harmful mutation can be overlooked and give rise to a cancer cell. Genetic mutations are found in nearly all types of cancer.

What causes these mutations in the first place? Some of them have genetic origins, from 'oncogenes' that have the potential to cause cancer. When researchers first started studying genes that could be linked to cancer, they found that there are numerous oncogenes and they are in all of us, always. It is important to emphasise that these are normal genes that are involved in deciding when cell division should occur. When they mutate however, they become hyperactive and tell the cell to continue dividing, with the production of more and more cells.

The researchers also discovered another type of gene – 'tumour suppressor genes' – that stop uninhibited cell division when it should not be occurring and also tell cells when it is time to bring programmed cell death into action.

If the oncogenes are mistakenly activated and if the tumour suppressor genes don't apply the brakes effectively, you will get too many cells developing, leading eventually to cancer.

If the researchers could identify a small number of genes that were the cause of bowel cancer, for example, they could create a drug that attacked the specific genetic mutation so that bowel cancer could be cured.

Unfortunately, it's not so simple.

A FRUITLESS SEARCH FOR THE SUPERDRUG

As part of the efforts to solve the cancer puzzle, two huge projects have been running during the past two decades. The first of these, The Human Genome Project (HGP), was started in 1990 with a budget of 3 billion dollars and was completed in 2003 with a detailed chart of about 30,000 genes. This information will play an important part in further research on cancer.

The second big project, The Cancer Genome Atlas (TCGA) was started in 2005 with the aim of revealing which mutations were distinctive of particular cancers, so that drugs could be made to measure to combat the mutations. 10,000 tumours would be investigated to identify the right mutations to attack with drugs.

The first reports were published in 2015. Had the researchers identified mutations that could usefully be targeted in future cancer treatments? They had indeed – over ten million of them. Moreover, there were thousands of different mutations in the same type of cancer, different mutations in the same tumour and different mutations in 'similar' tumours from the same patient

To produce tailor-made drugs for such an overwhelming mass of mutations would clearly be impossible. Many people consider the TCGA project to have been an enormous disappointment (not to say an enormous drain of money away from other projects), because it apparently produced so little benefit in relation to the investment.

On average, each individual cancer cell contains over 200 mutations. And that is just one cancer cell. A tumour contains numerous cells and an enormous number of mutations. Following the confusing results that the TCGA project produced, some researchers have begun to ask: Is it likely that all these mutations arise just by chance, as the somatic mutation theory claims?

Can there be something other than chance errors inducing the mutations? The question has led to renewed interest in alternative theories about the causes of cancer.

MITOCHONDRIA –
PROBLEMS IN THE
POWERHOUSE

The theory that appears to be closest to explaining what recent research shows, is that cancer is the result of problems in the mitochondria, the cells' powerhouses. Early in the twentieth century the Nobel prize winner Otto Warburg discovered a phenomenon common to nearly all cancer cells: the mitochondria in the cancer cells looked very different from those in healthy cells. Nearly all cancer cells contained damaged and non-functioning mitochondria. In healthy cells, the mitochondria were effective structures that generated energy from glucose and oxygen, but cancer cells were unable to use this method to generate energy. Instead, cancer cells used a very ancient method of generating energy that humans have inherited from an earlier phase of evolution: the fermentation of glucose.

According to this theory the mutations are not the cause of the disease but are a symptom of damage to the mitochondria. When the mitochondria are damaged they send a stream of messages to the cell nucleus calling for changes to the genes. This leads to mutations and instability in the structure and function of the genes. If this theory is correct, the treatment of cancer should be directed against the cancer cells' vulnerability in respect of energy generation, instead of attempting to create made-to-measure weapons against a multiplicity of random mutations.

There is also historical evidence indicating a connection between intra-cellular energy systems and cancer. The British did a lot of research in colonial times and were amazed by the absence of cancer among many folk groups in Africa and Asia. Doctors who were accustomed to diagnosing cancer at home in Britain reported that during a whole working career in Africa they hardly saw a single case of cancer.

We could say that life expectation in Africa at that time was so low that people didn't survive to the age at which they would have been at most risk from cancer. On the other hand, life expectation in Great Britain was not very impressive either. At the beginning of the twentieth century the average life expectation in the UK was under 50 years, which is less than the age at which we commonly expect cancer to appear.

In India, the doctors also found big differences between different parts of the country, depending on the local diet. Cancer was much more prevalent in the parts of the country where carbohydrates were a significant part of the diet.[10]

A bigger health study was carried out between 1898 and 1905 on the indigenous population in North America, at a time when most of the Native Americans still lived on a traditional diet from hunting and fishing. The study recorded that most of them appeared to have spectacularly good health and to live to a ripe old age. The numbers supported this, showing that within the indigenous population there were 224 centenarians per million men and 254 per million women. In contrast, the 'white' population had 3 centenarians per million men and 6 per million women. The researchers were also impressed by the total absence of chronic diseases. They were told about 'tumours' and were able to see several varieties of tumours which all appeared to be benign. They didn't come across a single clearly malignant tumour during the whole time of the study.

So researchers were already aware at that time that diet and physical activity might be key factors in the development of cancer. There must be something in our environment or our lifestyle that makes us so liable to these diseases. Increasing average life expectancy cannot possibly be the only explanation for the high incidence of cancer. In Norway the latest figures from the Institute of Public Health show that people are becoming older but are also becoming sicker, and that young people are becoming sick earlier.

Perhaps the answer to the problem of cancer is to be found in our past history. If we live and eat more like our forefathers, can we hope to reduce the frighteningly high incidence of cancer?

Applying the dietary theory, the treatment of cancer focuses on attacking the cancer cells' dependence on glucose. Without functioning mitochondria, cancer cells cannot generate energy in the normal way and they become dependent on large amounts of sugar. The core of 'metabolic therapy' consists of changes in diet *in addition to* the usual measures such as surgery, radiation and chemotherapy. Drugs can also be used to attack the cancer cells' altered metabolic system.

During my search for 'the truth' about cancer I soon came across a particularly interesting study:

Researchers in a laboratory removed the cell nuclei from cancer cells and implanted them in healthy cells from which the 'healthy' nuclei had been removed. The 'sick' nuclei contained damaged and mutated DNA, and the researchers expected that the healthy cells would change into cancer cells, in accordance with the somatic mutation theory. However, this didn't happen. The researchers couldn't understand it. So they proceeded to replace mitochondria in healthy cells with 'sick' mitochondria from cancer cells. The previously healthy cells rapidly changed into cancer cells.[11]

I started to question my previous ideas about cancer. Was cancer not caused by an accumulation of unhealthy mutations as I had been taught as a student? There is sound research pointing to other causes.[12] This research shows that change of diet is a vital part of the strategy to attack what is probably cancer's most important weak point, energy supply. After careful reading through much basic and convincing research I found it not difficult to resist sugary temptations.

My mantra became: 'Don't feed the tumour!'

I understood of course that the tumour couldn't be starved into submission. There will always be glucose available in the blood stream because the liver can produce glucose from other substances. The research shows, however, that tumours don't need to be starved completely to achieve results. Eating less carbohydrate is enough to be effective.

If the theory of cancer as a metabolic disease where the power-house inside the cell is damaged turns out to be correct, will the focus of cancer prevention change? Possibly not. Mitochondria are damaged by the same things we consider to be the explanation for the mutation theory: toxins, alcohol, viruses, radiation, unhealthy diet, obesity and in some cases, genes.

Treatment strategies, on the other hand, can be changed. Diet will be given a more important place. For some types of cancer a diet without any carbohydrate – a ketogenic diet – has shown promising results, especially for certain types of brain cancer. For other types of cancer, research indicates that reducing the calories in the diet causes tumours to shrink.

Might the search for a 'superdrug' to cure cancer eventually come to a successful conclusion? Or is the answer to be found in a different strategy: effective drugs, surgery if necessary and radiotherapy if appropriate; all combined with changes to diet and physical activity? It appears that in addition to having an independent effect, metabolic therapy can enhance the effect of traditional cancer treatments such as chemotherapy and radiation. Diet is important not only in prevention but also in treatment of cancer.

The somatic mutation theory has been the leading paradigm for several decades and the basis for massive investment of money. After repeated defeats on the research front, has the time perhaps come to question the validity of a theory which assumes that millions of different mutations can arise by accident? Whatever the theoretical basis, it appears that the importance of diet in the prevention of cancer has been under-estimated, when we see that 30 per cent of the risk of cancer is related to diet, and that diet is important in the treatment of cancer when it is diagnosed.

Research shows among other things that in the fight against cancer, changing diet in order to exploit the cancer's dependency on glucose is a wise move. Cancer is a hard foe, but energy production from glucose may be its Achilles heel.

TEN COMMON FEATURES OF CANCERS

Even though the causes of cancer cannot be established with certainty, cancer cells do have a number of features in common. In my own battle against cancer, I came across the respected but debated article 'Hallmarks of Cancer' from 2000 (revised in 2011). The authors describe the features that all types of cancer have in common.13

I studied the article carefully. Here were the real distinguishing features of cancer cells. If I knew these, I could work out their weak points. The authors had the same outlook as myself. They identified certain shared characteristics and sketched out how these features also contained vulnerabilities that could be exploited using appropriate medicines.

A part of the puzzle was falling into place. I would do the same, with different weapons: proper nutrition and physical activity. I understood that combining these measures with what the oncologists recommended offered great potential.

Common features of cancer

1) Continuous division. The signals telling the cell to divide don't stop. Instead, the cell continuously receives orders to go on dividing. In children and young people whose bodies are still growing, a high rate of cell division to create the organs of the body is normal. This process slows

when we become adult. Cancer cells somehow manage to accelerate the programme again.

2) Avoidance of growth inhibition As part of our natural defence system against cancer, cells receive signals telling them when to stop dividing. Cancer cells ignore these signals. A healthy cell can be given permission to divide a certain number of times, until it gets the signal to stop. A cancer cell ignores the order and goes on dividing.

3) Invisibility. Cancer cells find a way of 'flying under the radar' of the immunological defence force.

4) Endless cell division. Cancer cells can go on dividing for ever. We don't yet know how they achieve this. In laboratories, there are cancer cell cultures that have been growing continuously since the 1960s.

5) Use of inflammation. Cancer cells can create local inflammation in their immediate vicinity. This helps the cancer cells to spread.

6) Expansion. Cancer cells can invade underlying tissues and spread to other organs.

7) Establishing their own blood supply. Cancerous tumours are dependent on setting up supply lines in the form of blood vessels to provide them with the nutrition they need.

8) Failure to correct harmful mutations. Changes in genes and chromosomes occur all the time, but we have an effective repair system that detects and corrects nearly all the mistakes that occur. Mutations that are not detected and corrected can lead to cancer.

9) Avoidance of programmed cell death. When something has gone wrong with a cell, our immunological security system will usually prevent it from dividing and send it an order to self-destruct. This mechanism of programmed cell death is known as 'apoptosis.' Cancer cells have found a way of avoiding apoptosis.

10) Disordered intra-cellular metabolism. Cancer cells have a quite different way of generating energy from nutrients.

THE BATTLE BEGINS

I gradually began to realise that there really were useful things I could do to improve my own prognosis. I read everything I could find. There were some measures that appeared to merit being put into action early. I quickly started cutting down on sugar, for this seemed to be one of the most promising lines of attack. Then I gradually set about almost completely cutting out other carbohydrates (bread, pasta, rice, potatoes, anything with added sugar, etc.) and switching my diet as far as possible towards vegetables.

My next move was to try to eat food that combats inflammation. I understood early on that inflammation is an important factor in enabling cancer to spread.

So I began eating masses of green vegetables, olive oil and omega-3 fatty-acid supplements. I seasoned the food with turmeric and pepper and started drinking green tea with ginger. I cut out alcohol almost completely, apart from a glass of red wine occasionally with a meal.

I had been quite active and physically fit before, but I started including several spells of intensive training (four times four-interval training sessions a couple of times per week), and I tried to arrange four or five training sessions each week. Several sources recommend physical activity in the fight against cancer, preferably five times a week. This could for example be a half-hour walk, but there appeared to be even more to be gained from intensive physical activity.

I took plenty of sun, so that my vitamin D stayed at the summer level, to strengthen my immune defences.

I also took antioxidants daily in the form of berries. Blueberries and raspberries are both good sources of antioxidants and a welcome substitute for sugar.

As time went on I deployed a number of minor measures and set aside some unhealthy old habits. Little by little, the various measures I was taking began to become quite comprehensive. Each step became a habit that did not require a lot of energy or force of will.

I was under no illusion that blueberries alone would be able to cure me of cancer or that I would become healthier just by eating broccoli, but I had developed the firm belief which I still hold, that the daily combination of all these types of measures can be a deadly combination for the cancer cells.

And I knew that there was no available research on that hypothesis.

ATTACK FROM SEVERAL DIRECTIONS – THE KEY TO SUCCESS?

A s nobody has yet carried out a study of patients combining dietary and lifestyle adjustments in the way I was doing, I had to be both the project leader and the laboratory animal. Researchers and doctors will tell you that there is no good evidence that broccoli can be effective against cancer, even though there are many smaller studies that indicate an effect. They will probably claim that adapting diet and lifestyle is not worth the effort, because there is no documented evidence that it will affect the prognosis.

In a way, they are right. It is often impossible to demonstrate an effect for each individual measure. However, no specialist can say that the combination of dietary measures and fitness training *doesn't* work, for studies have never been done to show that either.

How can the combination
be so effective?

In theory, you would expect that two equally effective therapies would double the effectiveness of treatment. In many instances, however, we find that the treatment works even better than the expected double effect. This is known as synergy. Each measure increases the effectiveness of the other.

HIV – a death sentence commuted to a lifelong suspended sentence

When the AIDS epidemic began to spread in the 1980s, many people were worried and fearful. For a long time it remained uncertain how contagious the disease was, and the diagnosis was originally thought of as a death sentence. There was no treatment that could even slow the disease down effectively.

Then when researchers started experimenting with a combination of different drugs, a 'cocktail' of medicines, treatment started becoming effective. Each drug on its own gave little effect as the HIV virus mutated and adapted, but combing different drugs at the same time was often successful.

Nowadays, HIV is considered to be a disease that patients die with, not one that they die from – if they live in a country where effective treatment is available.

COMBINED TREATMENTS

C ancer researchers have always dreamed of finding the 'cure,' the drug that will finally obliterate cancer cells. The target has often seemed to be in sight, but disappointment has always followed.

Even the new immunotherapy drugs that sometimes have an almost unbelievably good effect to begin with, often lose their effect after several months. Like the HIV virus, cancer cells are able to mutate and adapt themselves to resist the treatment.

Modern cancer drugs are designed to be as target-orientated as possible, so that they effectively kill the cancer cells but allow healthy cells to survive, thereby producing fewer side-effects. Drugs of this type often target a particular factor in the process of cell division. Modern treatment regimens also combine drugs that are toxic to cancer cells in several different ways. This gives greater effect, but also greater side-effects.

Particular success has been achieved in the treatment of leukaemia in children. Between the 1960s and the 2000s, the number of children surviving acute lymphoblastic leukaemia rose from 10 per cent to 90 per cent. This was not primarily because of revolutionary new drugs, but rather the result of clever combination of the drugs available – the synergy effect.

Can you contribute ingredients to make a 'cocktail' of effective measures against cancer in addition to traditional treatment? The answer is 'Yes,' and the more measures we can combine, the more we can hope to achieve a synergic effect.

The strength of this approach raises your attack on cancer to another level. By removing a potentially harmful food and substituting a food that can help to fight the cancer you will have a doubly favourable effect. In addition, the foods that you have chosen as allies will have a combined effect. What's more, several of these measures have been shown to enhance the effect of traditional treatments such as radiotherapy and chemotherapy.[14]

Many natural substances are effective inhibitors of cancer, even when the disease is already well established. They often work by increasing the body's own capacity for detoxification of carcinogenic substances.

A combination of various natural substances that act against cancer in different ways is likely to be more effective than one nutrient alone in slowing the development of cancer.

Even though there is research indicating effectiveness of a single nutrient against cancer, it is often difficult to prove the effect. It is difficult to study food as a 'medicine.' How easy would it be to gather tens of thousands of similar cancer patients and give them exactly the same diet over a long period? Studies of this sort are obviously impractical on a large scale.

The absence of big clinical studies proving the effectiveness of a treatment measure does not however mean that we should ignore the smaller studies.

It is certainly true that blueberries can't cure cancer, for example, but what about blueberries as a small component among a number of other measures?

'It is tempting to say that you should eat broccoli,' said my empathetic and knowledgeable oncologist who has been following me up for two years, 'but I can't point to any large, randomised, controlled studies that prove it, and therefore I cannot recommend it.'

That started me thinking. Nor are there any large, controlled studies showing that it is dangerous to drive with worn tyres. Nevertheless, we hopefully change our tyres before it is too late. I have neither time nor patience to wait until the big broccoli studies are available, but I have found many convincing smaller studies which indicate that eating broccoli is a smart move. So I choose to do it regularly.

PART 2:
EFFECTIVE STRATEGIES TO IMPROVE YOUR OWN PROGNOSIS

I continued my exploration of the literature. Reading about what cancer really is and what can influence the course of the disease made me more and more optimistic. I obviously didn't believe that I could be cured just by eating berries or vegetables; that would have been naïve. But it did appear that I could influence the progress of the disease and buy myself more time.

I had emphatically accepted that I was not invulnerable and invincible, even if I had ever thought of myself so. At the same time, I also understood that neither were cancer cells totally invincible. That gave me a certain confidence.

I realised that even though each individual move I made would probably not save me, nobody could know the potential of combining a range of large and small measures. That was what I would find out.

Bad luck, circumstances and perhaps an unsound diet had been steering my health in the wrong direction for many years, and the result was cancer. I would try to turn things round. With the help of diet and fitness training, could I turn the situation to my own advantage and to the cancer cells' disadvantage?

The following pages deal with how we can make use of the cancer cell's weak points, for example its total dependence on a good blood supply to be able to grow. Without a blood supply, a cancerous tumour won't manage to grow bigger than a snowflake.

STRATEGY 1:

*Eat food that damages the
cancer cells' blood supply*

A cancerous tumour cannot grow bigger unless it has a good blood supply. The tumour deceives the body into creating new blood vessels, a process that is otherwise tightly regulated. Certain foods can help us to slow down or even cut off the tumour's blood supply. Hindering the blood supply is one of many ways in which choice of diet can be useful.

About blood supply

The body contains a network of several billion blood vessels, that would stretch twice round the world if laid out end to end. No cell can survive without contact with the blood circulation. Nutrients and oxygen are transported to the cell and waste materials from the cell's metabolism are carried away.

In an adult human, new blood vessels are not usually created, except as part of the repair process of wounds or other injuries. This process is strictly controlled. When the body signals the need for new vessels, proteins are produced which initiate their creation. As soon as the need has been met, inhibitors are produced which halt the manufacture.

Faults arising in this process can lead to illness. The most serious is when cancer cells hijack the system for their own benefit, to acquire the supplies they need. Without a new blood supply, a tumour cannot grow bigger than half a cubic millimetre and without access to the blood circulation, cancer cells cannot spread throughout the body.

Most of us probably have numerous microscopic cancer tumours in various organs. A study in the USA investigated people who had died in traffic accidents. The results showed that 40 per cent of women aged 40 – 50 had microscopic tumours in their breasts and about 50 per cent of men between 50 and 60 had microscopic tumours in their prostate glands.[15] Fortunately, most of these cancer cells don't develop any further. Without a dedicated blood supply they remain microscopic and are made harmless by the body's defence mechanisms.

The inhibition of new blood vessel creation is one of the reasons these cancer cells don't grow to become dangerous. An example from a big American study shows how regular intake of cooked tomatoes reduces the risk of cancer and helps people who already have cancer.[16]

How you can do it

Many types of food can help to reduce the creation of new blood vessels. The effect of substances within these foods in impeding blood vessel formation has been compared with the effect of drugs. Some nutrients were found to be as good or almost as good as the drugs in this respect.[17] Combining several of the foodstuffs can further increase the effect.

Foods that help to inhibit new blood vessel formation include:

Apples
Blackberries
Blueberries
Cabbage
Sea cucumber
Garlic
Ginseng
Grape juice
Grapefruit
Green tea
Lavender
Lemons
Liquorice
Maitake mushrooms
Dark chocolate
Olive oil
Oranges
Parsley
Pineapples
Pumpkins
Raspberries
Red grapes

Red wine
Nutmeg
Soya beans
Strawberries
Tomatoes
Tuna fish
Turmeric

Amounts

Regular intake is beneficial, but variety is also important for the combined effect of different nutrients. A cupful of berries every day is recommended. A couple of squares of dark chocolate every day can also have a positive effect. A glass of red wine low on sugar may be taken several times a week, along with food so that it doesn't increase the blood sugar too much. It's important to drink green tea often; studies have shown good effects from 3 – 5 cups per day.[18]

The vegetables can be taken with the main meal of the day, but the addition of a couple of cloves of garlic per day can also be helpful. Turmeric can be sprinkled over the food (half to one teaspoonful). Ground black pepper significantly increases the absorption of turmeric.[19]

Many of the foods on the list may already be part of your diet, but by taking a systematic approach to check that they are part of your *daily* meals you will get a good ally in your attack on the cancer's supply lines. You can also find further practical tips and advice about good anti-cancer diet in Part 3.

Remember!
The creation of new blood vessels is essential for cancer tumours to be able to grow, but can be reduced with the help of nutrients in a number of foods.

STRATEGY 2:

*Avoid and clear out
damaging substances*

Pollutants in the environment can lead to cancer. It should be just as important to think about these even after cancer has been diagnosed and confirmed. Whatever causes cancer to start can probably also make the disease worse. Sometimes I was tempted to think the opposite: 'It's too late now, there's no longer any point in avoiding unhealthy things.' However, my will to live generally won in the end. The inner voice telling me that I must try to make life hard for the cancer cells was stronger.

Cancer cells flourish in a milieu where healthy cells don't. Tobacco, alcohol, toxins in food and pollutants in the environment can lead to an unhealthy internal milieu. My aim would have to be to eliminate risk factors in order to improve my chances.

The unanswered question of why I had got cancer in the first place bothered me. Throughout my life I had assumed that I was living healthily. As a medical student I had been particularly concerned to lead a good lifestyle, scared by all the diseases I was learning about. The lecturers told us about the toxins that damage cellular DNA and lead to harmful mutations that promote cancer. They listed smoking, alcohol, environmental toxins, air pollution, chemicals, excessive sun, radiation and some types of viruses. The mantra that we were taught most emphatically was to encourage the patients to 'Stop smoking!'

I suspect many people are tired of doctors nagging them to stop smoking, and I have come to realise that we need to work together to achieve the necessary motivation. The doctor's warning finger seldom works. Many people find it very difficult to stop smoking without strong inner motivation. Exposing the relationship between tobacco and all types of cancer – not just lung cancer – may help motivation.

The toxins we are exposed to

Modern research has produced much evidence to underline the fact that if the body's cells are exposed to toxins – such as tobacco – over a long time, cells become damaged. This can lead to mutations and cancer.

Excessive alcohol use can have the same effects. Alcohol is particularly associated with cancer in the mouth, throat, oesophagus, liver, breast and large bowel. An American study from 2009 showed that alcohol was implicated in 3.5 per cent of deaths from cancer.[20] Alcohol is broken down in the liver to acetaldehyde, which is toxic and can damage the cells. In the process of breaking it down further, harmful reactive oxidants are also produced. Alcohol also has the effect of reducing the body's capacity to utilise nutrients that can hinder cancer growth, such as vitamins C, D and E.

Numerous other toxic substances can have similar destructive effects to tobacco and alcohol.

How you can do it

There are two aspects to consider. One is substances you should not ingest, inhale or otherwise take in. The other is foodstuffs you should make part of your daily diet to eliminate harmful materials.

It is important to stop smoking. If you think this is difficult, you can ask your doctor for help. Some people benefit from tablets, patches, courses or other measures. However, the most important thing is for you to decide to stop and consider that the pain of stopping is a price worth paying for the profit in health. One method is to reduce by one cigarette per day until daily consumption is zero. If you smoke ten per day, for example, this would take just ten days.

Cut down on alcohol, but a glass of red wine with a meal is OK. Preferably choose a dry wine with as little sugar as possible (preferably less than 5 grams per litre). Red wine is advised because it contains the beneficial substance resveratrol plus useful antioxidants.

Antioxidants can neutralise harmful free radicals
Free radicals are strongly reactive chemicals that have the potential to damage our cells. Radiation and environmental pollutants are among the things that can cause abnormally high concentrations of free radicals in the body. When a cancer tumour is treated with radiotherapy, one of the ways the radiotherapy works is by creating large amounts of free radicals, which kill the cancer cells. Antioxidants work alongside the free radicals against the cancer cells, but they also neutralise free radicals to restrict the treatment from damaging health cells. Fruit and berries are rich in antioxidants.

As far as possible, try to avoid potentially harmful chemicals which are known or suspected to be carcinogenic. These include:

Insecticides
Chemical sprays. Preferably eat organic food that has not been exposed to agricultural sprays.
Chemical cleaning products, including chemical car-cleaning products. Look for cleaning products that don't contain alkylphenols. Use organic products, green soap, sodium bicarbonate or vinegar.
Cosmetics containing parabens or phthalates. Organic cosmetics are free of these.

Deodorants containing aluminium.
Perfumes containing phthalates.
PVC plastics: Many drink containers, food boxes and cartons contain PVC plastics that can seep into food and drink when heated. It is better to warm things up in glass or ceramic containers.
Teflon-lined pans that have been scratched, if made before 2014 when new regulations came into force.

As most parts of our environment contain potentially toxic substances, it is impossible to avoid contact with them in one form or another. Therefore, your diet should include food and drink that counteracts them.

Green tea acts as a detoxicant, by activating processes in the liver to eliminate toxins more effectively. Animal studies have shown how green tea blocks the effects of chemical toxins that are associated with cancers of the breast, lung, oesophagus, stomach and large bowel.[21]

Strawberries, raspberries and nuts have similar beneficial effects to green tea because of their content of ellagic acid which blocks the transformation of environmental toxins into harmful substances.

Cherries contain gluconic acid which can lead to toxic substances being converted into non-dangerous compounds.[22]

Remember!
Avoid toxins such as tobacco, excessive alcohol intake and harmful chemicals. Preferably, choose organically grown food so as to avoid vegetables and fruit that have been exposed to agricultural chemicals. As it is almost impossible to avoid potential toxins in one form or another in our modern diet, your daily intake should include food and drink that act against them.

STRATEGY 3:

Reduce stress

My life as a father of young children and a busy doctor was sometimes chaotic. It is now almost impossible to look back on these very busy times, because I can't understand how I managed to live with constant stress, little sleep and heavy responsibilities every day for so many years.

Why hadn't I taken some important steps earlier to reduce the stress in my life?

I think it was because I saw it as normal; that's how it was for everybody; life was like that. It was only when I had made changes to my life and emerged from this 'stress-bubble' that I was able to see the folly of it all. The diagnosis of cancer was the warning shot I needed to make me change course.

Stress increases the level of stress hormones. This can be beneficial in the short term, but if continued it is harmful in the long term. Chronic stress with increased hormone levels over a long time weakens the immune system that is so important to us in fighting cancer and other diseases. Can you reduce stress to give your immune system better working conditions and yourself a better daily life?

Many people who are diagnosed with cancer are struck with a feeling of helplessness. You lose control over your own health, and it is easy to be overwhelmed by fears of a future that has suddenly become more uncertain and sinister. Your attitude is further disturbed by previous experiences and stories of the effects of cancer.

I eventually realised that I would need to get a grip of my stress level. I was fortunate in being able to cut down on my work. I was released from out-of-hours and nursing home duties and was able to concentrate fully on the patients on my GP list. This gave me time and energy for regular physical activity, which further reduced my stress levels. I chose to step away from optional management duties in favour of spending more time with my family.

Such measures can seem difficult to carry through when you are in the middle of it all, but I think you rarely regret them afterwards. By creating more calm – more quality – in your own life, you can strengthen your immunological defences and probably also your quality of life. These can build up your capacity to meet the challenges that lie ahead.

Stress

Stress hormones are useful to us in an acute, threatening situation. They help us to mobilise the resources needed for 'fight or flight.' Adrenalin, noradrenaline and cortisol increase alertness and reaction speed. The pulse beats faster, breathing speeds up, the blood carries more oxygen to the muscles, the senses are sharpened.

However, these potentially life-saving stress hormones become dangerous if the levels are kept high, as happens if you live under stressful circumstances for a long time. Chronic stress has several adverse effects on your health.

High levels of stress hormones weaken the immune system. You may have noticed that you are more at risk of catching infections in times of stress. Studies have shown that high levels of stress hormones make the immune system less effective against cancer cells in the breast, ovary or prostate gland.[23] Stress also drains energy from us, which makes living a healthy, active lifestyle more difficult. When you are under constant stress, it is easy to fall into bad habits such as poor diet, physical inactivity, smoking and increased alcohol intake.

It is not just excessive commitments and overpacked schedules of work and daily life that cause stress. Emotional challenges such as conflicts, grief, worries and feelings of helplessness also increase the stress level.

A point that is seldom mentioned in discussions about cancer is that a persistent feeling of helplessness increases the level of the stress hormone, noradrenaline, which in turn leads to an increase production of inflammatory factors in anticipation of a need to repair possible injury. As strategy five will show, cancer cells can use inflammation to divide and spread more easily. So it is important to keep the substances involved in the immune response to a minimum level.[24] This may be why some anti-inflammatory drugs such as ibuprofen, naproxen and diclofenac have been shown to have some effect in preventing or limiting cancer.[25] Because of undesirable side-effects, however, these drugs are not recommended for cancer treatment.

How you can do it

What can you do to reduce the stress level in your life? Think how to prioritise your time. Get a grip on your schedule if you can. Seek help from friends and family if you can. Cut out unnecessarily energy- and time-consuming obligations. Even though it might feel selfish at the moment, the reserves of time and energy you can achieve may make you able to give more back later.

Make use of relaxation techniques. Learn yoga, mindfulness or other methods. (See page ..... for suggestions.) Can you learn to worry less? Consider seeking professional help such as cognitive therapy from a counsellor, psychologist or psychiatrist.

Sharing the responsibility for your own treatment regimen can give you a feeling of regaining control of your own destiny.

Remember!
Raised levels of stress hormones can reduce your immune defences.
Keep the stress hormones down by removing unnecessary activities
from your daily routine.

STRATEGY 4:

*Reduce excessive hormone
levels and obesity*

I used to love bread, pizza and everything sweet. I would eat big portions of pasta after exercise, keen to build up the glycogen stores in my muscles after a training session. Carbohydrates are super food if you aim is to build up the body. In response to the excess of sugar provided by carbohydrates, the body produces anabolic hormones that promote growth.

Unfortunately, it is not only our healthy cells that are influenced by the growth-promoting hormones; cancer tumours will also be stimulated to grow. To tell the truth, I still love carbohydrates, but the knowledge that the anabolic hormones insulin and IGF-1 (insulin-like growth factor 1) promote tumour growth makes it easier now for me to avoid them. I realised that cutting down carbohydrate in the diet, losing weight and physical activity can help to reduce the levels of these hormones.

Hormones

Hormones are produced in various glands and function as 'messengers' that initiate and regulate various processes in the body. The relationship between raised levels of certain hormones and cancer is well known. Hormones such as insulin, IGF-1, oestrogen and leptin can all stimulate tumour growth.

When the level of sugar in the blood rises, insulin is secreted. The hormone facilitates the uptake of sugar from the blood stream into the cells, which use the sugar as fuel. Insulin also acts as a growth hormone. It stimulates growth when there is good access to the necessary nutrients. Cancer cells can make good use of this.

A 500 ml. bottler of a sugary soft drink can contain as much as 50 grams of sugar, equivalent to about 25 sugar cubes. When you drink this the blood sugar level rises fast and insulin is secreted in response. It doesn't take very much for the insulin level to become too high, and if this happens several times a day you can almost be sure that the raised insulin level will benefit the cancer cells and act to your disadvantage.

Insulin also acts as a growth hormone, stimulating growth when nutrients are readily available. Cancer cells make use of this.

Foodstuffs containing mostly protein and fat mobilise insulin to a small extent, but foodstuffs rich in carbohydrate cause insulin to flood into the bloodstream. However, not all carbohydrates are the same. Some types, such as highly refined wheat in buns, cause a rapid rise in blood sugar, whereas others, such as less refined cereals in wholemeal bread, cause a slower rise. One method of describing how big a sugar load you are taking on and therefore the amount of insulin that will be secreted, is what is known as the glycaemic index (see fact-box later in this chapter for details). A high glycaemic index indicates a large sugar load and consequent high insulin secretion.

People who are overweight often have high levels of insulin and IGF-1. Both of these hormones lead to increase of inflammatory factors and thereby to growth and spread of cancer (see also Strategy 5).[26] There is well documented evidence that both obesity and diabetes increase the risk of at least thirteen types of cancer.[27] These types of cancer accounted for 40 per cent of all new diagnoses of cancer in 2014. The cancer risk associated with obesity rises drastically with every extra kilogram of body weight. For example, if an adult woman puts on an extra 5 kg. of body weight, her risk of breast cancer rises by 11 per cent. Increased weight implies an increase in stored body fat. Fatty tissue produces oestrogen, which is associated with breast, ovarian, uterine and other cancers. It also produces leptin, which is thought to stimulate cell division.

The insulin level is not only important in relation to growth of the cancer. It is also the key to controlling body weight. One of the insulin hormone's functions is to help the body to store energy sources for use later. If the laying down of energy reserves is turned on, the fat cells grow and the kilos mount up.

As it is only carbohydrates that raise the blood sugar level and stimulate insulin secretion, it is probable that excessive dietary carbohydrate is the main reason why western populations are becoming more and more overweight. Statistics from the 1970s to today show that fat intake has fallen from over 40% of our diet in the 1970s to about 30 per cent today. This has happened because of advice to reduce fat intake to avoid cardiovascular disease. At the same time, the weight increase in the population has exploded. Why? The fat removed from the diet has had to be substituted by something else. That 'something else' has largely been carbohydrates.

By following the advice to reduce our fat intake, we have taken away a nutrient that doesn't affect blood sugar and insulin levels and replaced it with a nutrient that does. By doing this, we have laid the foundations for weight increase and increased the prevalence of life-style related diseases.

In addition to carbohydrate reduction and losing weight, physical activity is another key to maintaining a normal and beneficial hormone balance. For example, exercise reduces the oestrogen level.[28] Exercise also helps to reduce the blood sugar levels and therefore the secretion of insulin and the IGF-1 growth hormone.

We need insulin to live, but the problem arises when the

insulin level is too high over a period of time. Raised insulin levels are associated with both overweight and cancer.[30] Insulin can stimulate the cancer cells to grow. It is important to note that what is important is not necessarily the amount of food, but whether the ingredients lead to high insulin levels.[31]

How you can do it

It is only the carbohydrates that cause significant rises in blood sugar and increased secretion of insulin and IGF-1.[32] Avoid having too much carbohydrate in your diet, in order to keep the hormone levels low.

First, eliminate the carbohydrates that cause the fastest increase in blood sugar: sweet foods such as chocolate, cakes, sugary drinks and so on. We are often advised to drink apple juice without added sugar, but that contains up to 100 grams of sugar per litre, equivalent to about 50 sugar cubes.

Vegetables can replace pasta and rice to reduce the quantity of carbohydrates further. You can take vegetables freely, except for potatoes and maize which are rich in glucose. Choose broccoli or other green vegetables instead of potatoes with your main meal. Broccoli contains about 0.8 grams of glucose per portion, as compared with 36 grams of glucose in a portion of potatoes.

Choose coarse rather than fine bread, or even better: do without bread. An intermediate measure, or a first step towards doing without bread completely, can be protein bread or home baked low carbohydrate bread. A slice of wholemeal bread contains about 22 grams of glucose (= 11 sugar cubes).

All the members of the onion family help to control the blood sugar level. That lowers production of insulin and IGF-1, and thereby reduces cancer growth.

Glycaemic index
The glycaemic index (GI) is a measure of how quickly carbohydrates are

broken down into sugars in the small intestine. Foodstuffs with a high GI are broken down quickly, leading to a rapid rise in the blood sugar. Foods with a lower GI take longer to break down and keep the blood sugar level more stable.

Fat and fibre slow absorption. So if you include some 'healthy' fat in a meal that includes carbohydrates with a high GI, the GI of the meal as a whole will be reduced.

Classification of foods by glycaemic index

Low GI (<55)
Milk without added flavours
All types of yoghurt
Wholemeal bread
Pumpernickel bread
Spaghetti and macaroni, cooked *al dente*
Noodles, *al dente*
Brown or wholegrain rice
Orange juice and apple juice
Oranges, apples, pears, grapes, kiwi fruit, peaches and mangos
Strawberries

Raw carrot, cucumber, paprika, maize and tomatoes
Lentils and beans (boiled)
All types of nuts
Dark chocolate

Medium GI (56-69)
Porridge
Wholemeal crispbread
Semi-refined bread
Spelt bread
Oatcakes
Mixed grains, rice (basmati, jasmine), couscous
Tacos shells, nachos
Popcorn
Bananas, pineapples
Raisins

High GI (>70)
Fine bread
Fine baguettes, rolls, wheaten buns
Croissants

Waffles
Wheat meal
Rice cakes
Cornflakes, refined breakfast cereals
Fast-boil rice
Potatoes (Boiled or baked)
Mashed potatoes (whether from whole potatoes or powder)
Boiled carrots or swedes
Watermelon
Sports drinks

Remember!
Restrict the amount of carbohydrates in your diet and be physically active. That will help you to avoid high hormone levels and obesity, which can stimulate tumour growth.

STRATEGY 5:

Reduce inflammation

One thought which constantly worried me was that the cancer had found its way to spread to other parts of my body. The link between inflammation and cancer spread was a common theme in the literature I was working my way through. Inflammation appeared to be a decisive factor that could enable the cancer to win. If I could suppress the inflammatory processes in my own body, would that help to swing the balance in my favour?

Inflammation makes it easier for cancer tumours to grow and spread, and can also play a part in cancer starting. You can play your part in preventing or slowing cancer by avoiding toxins and food that stimulate inflammation and eating food that has an anti-inflammatory effect.

Inflammation is a useful natural process, but it can become dangerous, rather like over-enthusiastic repair attempts causing a house to collapse.

Inflammation

Most of us have experienced inflammation at one time or another. It can arise as a response to invading bacteria or viruses, or as a response to injury such as around a strained tendon for example. Sometimes it can be part of an 'auto-immune' disease where the immune system somehow reacts against the body's own tissues instead of just against alien invaders.

Inflammation is part of a process of repair of bodily tissue. Important agents in this process are the white blood cells – the immune system's white knights who patrol the body, challenging invaders and helping to repair breeches in the defence.

We also recognise a distinction between acute inflammation that lasts for a few hours or days, and chronic inflammation that can continue for months or years. Acute inflammation is important in wound repair. Chronic inflammation, however, can be harmful. This can arise if you are exposed to injurious substances over a long period. Examples include: tobacco smoke; harmful chemicals; longstanding raised insulin levels; or chronic infections such as hepatitis C, Helicobacter Pylori or human papillomavirus. Chronically raised insulin levels can result either from insulin intolerance or from excessive carbohydrates in the diet. Chronic inflammation injures healthy cells and weakens the immune system.[34]

The role of inflammation in the development and progression of cancer is the result of a 'well-intentioned' attempt by the body's defence systems to repair damage. Unfortunately, the cancer cells find cunning ways to turn to their advantage the weapons that are directed against them. In normal wound healing, the increased production of inflammatory factors stops as soon as the wound is healed. In cancer, however, the outpouring of these substances continues. This excess leads to the programme of natural, programmed cell death ('apoptosis') being suspended. All cells start life programmed to commit suicide if they start to divide inappropriately. This mechanism is switched off if there are too many inflammatory factors in the vicinity, because wounds in the process of healing require a supply of fresh cells, produced by cell-division. In the absence of the programmed cell death mechanism, the cancer tumour secures its own survival, enabling it to grow and expand into neighbouring areas. Wherever the cancer spreads, it stimulates further inflammation around itself and achieves further growth.

Over-production of inflammatory factors appears to have yet another catastrophic effect: the white blood cells that should be protecting the body against unwelcome invaders are 'blinded' and no longer able to recognise and pick out the cancer cells.[35]

In some instances, inflammation is present in the earliest phases of the development of cancer. Researchers have shown that inflammation is essential for the development of cancer cells from an early phase to full-blown disease.[36] Therefore, inappropriate inflammation must be suppressed.

How you can do it

Restrict or avoid unhealthy foods and choose healthy foods instead. Try to lose excess weight and be physically active. Eat foods that reduce inflammation, such as asparagus, broccoli, chilli peppers, kale, paprika, pumpkin, root ginger, spinach, squash, sweet potato, turnip and other vegetables.

Put more vegetables on your plate. Aim for ¾ of your food to be vegetables and ¼ proteins and fats from meat, fish, chicken or egg. Try to choose products from free-grazing and hormone-free animals and wild-caught fish. Farm-grown fish often have an excess of omega-6 in relation to omega-3 fatty acids. By eating the smaller types of oily fish such as sardines, herring and mackerel you can also avoid the risk of accumulating heavy metals which can be present in larger fish. Select pure natural yoghurt and kefir without added sugar.

Benefit from anti-inflammatory supplements such as turmeric, pepper, green tea, ginger and foods rich in omega-3.

Avoid foods with a high ratio of omega-6 in relation to omega-3 fatty acids. The end-products of the metabolism of omega-6 acids appear to promote inflammation in several ways, in contrast to omega-3 acids which have the opposite effect. Good sources of omega-3 fatty acids include avocado, chia seeds, halibut, pecan nuts, salmon, tuna and walnuts. Prefer cooking oils with high omega-3 content such as olive oil and rapeseed oil, rather than corn-, sunflower- or soya oils with their omega-6 content.

It is also worthwhile to restrict your use of processed foods, which contain fewer nutrients and more highly refined sugars and cereals. Especially avoid highly processed items such as fast food and ready-made meals. Restrict your intake of processed meat such as bacon, sausages and pepperoni. Avoid sugary soft drinks and sports drinks, and minimise your alcohol intake.

Strategies 4, 7 and 8 can also help to combat inflammation.

Omega-3 and omega-6 fatty acids
Try to have a good balance between your intake of omega-3 and omega-6 fatty acids. Omega-6 stimulates cell growth, inflammation and blood clotting. Omega-3 works the opposite way to control cell growth, suppress inflammation and reduce blood clotting. Eating too many processed foods can give you more omega-6 than omega-3, resulting in an increased tendency to inflammation and cell growth, from which the cancer cells can benefit.[37]

Remember!
Prolonged inflammation injures the body's healthy cells and tissues and weakens the immune system. This not only increases the risk of cancer but also gives it better growing conditions. Avoid pro-inflammatory factors and eat anti-inflammatory foods.

STRATEGY 6:

Boost immune defences

T hinking about my cancer sometimes made me angry. I wanted to clench my fists and hit back against it. A feeling of helplessness was the trigger for my short-lived anger. The thought that I had no effective weapon against the invisible intruder was depressing.

However, I was not in fact totally defenceless. All my life, my immune system had been protecting me from potentially dangerous infections and killing off abnormal cells. Was there some way I could reinforce my immune defences to fight the cancer?

Your immune system rescues you from potentially dangerous infections every day. You are also entirely dependent on it to restrict and combat an established cancer. New cancer drugs mobilise the immune system's ability to kill cancer cells ('immunotherapy'). Physical activity, vitamins and the right food all maximise the effectiveness of the immune defences.

The first time I read about the many and indispensable actions of vitamin D, I was amazed. A team of researchers was observing a tuberculosis bacterium under a microscope, to study how the immune cells attacked it. However, no matter what the researchers tried the immune cells did nothing at all. By chance, the scientists discovered that there was something lacking in the serum where the battle was being staged – vitamin D. As soon as vitamin D was added, the immune cells started growing 'weapons' on their surface and slaughtering the bacterium.

The researchers soon worked out how the vitamin had helped the immune cells. Vitamin D worked as a key to open up the 'library' of DNA within the cells. The library contained the formulae the cells needed to do their job. Without the key to this information, the immune cells were helpless.

Immune defences

Our immune systems are constantly defending us against unwanted micro-organisms.

The immune system also kills cells that have arisen by mistake, for example by abnormal cell division. Cancer, however, has ways of neutralising the immune defences.

In someone with cancer, the immune cells often fail to react to damaged DNA or mutations in the cancer cells. One reason for this is that the patient's immune cells have developed alongside the cancer cells over a long period of time and appear to have become 'blind' to the harmful cancer cells. The cancer cells also create molecules that switch the immune cells off.

Front-line immune defence forces require supplies of vitamins such as B, C, D, E and K, plus reinforcements provided by physical activity and absence of stress. A vitamin is a substance that the body requires but cannot manufacture itself. Vitamin D, 'the sunshine vitamin,' is very important for the immune system and is unusual in that the body can manufacture it using energy from sunlight. We receive 80-90% of our vitamin D from exposure to sunlight. In countries with long, dark winters it may be necessary to take supplements or cod-liver oil during parts of the year.

One of the functions of **vitamin D** is to suppress unwanted cell division. It works as a bridge-builder, establishing connections between our cells. Cells that are linked together have less tendency to uninhibited cell division than cells that are unattached. Members of a 'community' of cells receive cautionary signals from their neighbours. An isolated cell receives fewer correcting signals and is more likely to start uninhibited division.

So it is important to have enough vitamin D for its controlling effect on cell division and its stimulant effect on the immune system.

People in countries in high latitudes, such as Norway, have lower average levels of vitamin D as compared with countries that have sunshine during more months each year. Norway is also among the countries with high incidences of bowel cancer and breast cancer, and it has been suggested that there may be a causal relationship with vitamin D levels. Sunshine playing on your skin not only helps to synthesise vitamin D but also generates a hormone, beta endorphin, that helps you to relax, dulls pain and kills newly generated cancer cells.

Vitamin C supports various cellular functions in the immune system, and also has a powerful antioxidant effect. It appears to increase the number and effectiveness of white blood cells, probably by its effect in regulating genes.

Vitamin C is already used in cancer treatment to enhance the effect of some cytotoxic anti-cancer drugs. Studies of liver cancer have shown a dramatic effect of vitamin C in restricting cancer cell growth and destroying liver cancer cells.[38]

The fat-soluble **vitamins K$_1$ and K$_2$** are present especially in green-leaf vegetables, cooking oils and well-matured cheeses. Studies from as far back as the 1950s indicate that vitamin K can restrict cancer and enhance the effect of some cytotoxic drugs. A Japanese study in 2004 showed that Japanese women who took vitamin K$_2$ for its anti-inflammatory effect had a 90% reduced risk of liver cancer.[39] Another study of liver cancer showed a 30% reduced risk of relapse in patients who took vitamin K$_2$ for three years after completing the initial treatment.[40]

The **E vitamins** include a group known as tocotrienols,

which have antioxidant effects. Laboratory and animal studies have demonstrated the effectiveness of vitamin E in restricting cell growth and regulating cell division by promoting the death of cancer cells and limiting the creation of new blood vessels.[41]

Some species of mushroom can also stimulate immune defence. Japanese mushrooms such as shitake, maitake, karawatake and enokitake contain a molecule called lentinan. Together with other substances present in the mushroom, this stimulates the immune system directly.

How you can do it

Make sure that you have the necessary vitamins, especially those that are important in building up your immune defences.

Sources of vitamins
Vitamin C: Fruit, especially citrus and kiwi fruit; berries such as strawberries, blackcurrants and rose-hips; paprika; broccoli; swede; spinach; tomato.
Vitamin D: Sunshine; fish; fish oils (including cod-liver oil).
Vitamin E: Walnuts; pine kernels; cloudberries; sunflower seeds; lingonberries; dandelion; paprika; almonds.
Vitamin K: The richest sources of vitamin K_2 are liver and well-matured cheese. Vitamin K is also created by fermentation of vegetables, and fermented soya beans are a particularly good source of vitamin K_2. Most of the studies referred to have used vitamin K in doses of up to 45 mg. per day. If you are taking anticoagulant drugs, it is important to check with your doctor whether it is safe to take extra vitamin K, because of its effect on blood clotting.

Are dietary supplements effective?

Professional opinion is divided about the effectiveness of dietary supplements. If you take sufficient of the necessary vitamins and minerals in a healthy diet, supplements will be unnecessary, with the possible exception in Northerly latitudes of taking cod-liver oil or other vitamin D supplements during the dark months of autumn and winter.

The possible benefits of vitamin C, multivitamin or other supplements are more debatable. Some large studies have shown that taking vitamin pills can have adverse rather than beneficial effects on health.

The reason for these surprising and disappointing results is that the dietary supplementation has not reproduced the effects of the vitamins in laboratory investigations.[42] One common interpretation of this is that the vitamins do have a positive effect but that it is probably more effective to absorb vitamins and minerals as part of a comprehensive, healthy diet that gives you the benefit of all the nutrients acting together.

We also know that the content of vitamins and minerals in the food we eat is lower than it was a few decades ago, largely because of new agricultural methods and genetic modification. Reports from health authorities show, among other things, that the intake of vitamin E, for example, is about half of the optimal recommended level. Because the authorities do not foresee serious consequences from this, however, they do not recommend supplements. Nevertheless, vitamin E has important roles in immune defence. The statistics also show that levels of vitamin K are also often less than optimal.

Another point worth noting is that 'normal' doesn't necessarily imply 'optimal.' The quantity of a vitamin in the body can be measured by a blood test, but what is a 'normal' level? Most laboratories quote a normal reference range for vitamin D of between 50-150 nmol/l. All this means is that 95% of the local population have levels within this range. So if your doctor tells you that you have a level of 55 nmol/l, all this means is that you are within the 'normal' range. It doesn't necessarily mean that you have an optimal amount of vitamin D in your body.

In comparison, a laboratory in Kenya could quote a 'normal range' between 100-175 nmol/l, because the population in Kenya on average have a much higher level than a Northern European population. The average vitamin D level is Kenya is about 110 nmol/l, as compared with about 50 nmol/l in Norway. Professor Johan Moan at the Radium Hospital in Oslo has been researching vitamin D for years. He recommends that people in Norway should try to maintain all year round a summer level of vitamin D, about 100 nmol/l.

Therefore, you should not be satisfied with a vitamin D level of 50 nmol/l. All this means is that you have just as inadequate vitamin D stores as most other people living in countries with short sunny seasons.

Another point is that when expert panels make recommendations about dietary content of vitamins, their criterion is what level is necessary to avoid deficiency diseases. Taking vitamin D as an example again, a serious shortage can lead to weakness and deformity of the bones; rickets in children or 'adult rickets' (osteomalacia) in older people. The current recommended intake is calculated to avoid this but says nothing about what level would be best for health generally.

Similarly, recommendations for vitamin C are calculated to avoid the serious vitamin deficiency disease of scurvy but say nothing about what is really best for health, for example with cancer prevention in mind.

It is commonly claimed that you will get all you need from a normal healthy diet. But what is a 'normal healthy diet?' Some of my patients tell me that they have a normal Norwegian diet when most of what they eat is plant-based, whereas others eat mainly pizza and tacos and consider that as normal. A person who eats a healthy, varied diet, cooks from raw ingredients and resists the temptation of ready-meals obviously has less need of supplements than somebody who eats a lot of fast-food.

My own recommendation is first and foremost to eat the best possible diet, with plenty of vegetables, fish, eggs, nuts, berries and olive oil. Buy cod-liver oil and omega-3 supplements preferably from a quality supplier.

Personally, I try to get exposure to sunlight all year

round, without becoming sunburnt. I follow Professor Johan Moan's advice to sunbathe preferably before noon, when the sun stimulates most vitamin D synthesis and causes least damage to the skin. In winter I try to have ten minutes per week in a solarium, and I take vitamin D supplements. I get vitamin C from my diet, and especially from eating berries every day.

Almonds are a rich source of vitamin E, and also of magnesium. Getting enough vitamin K can be a challenge, but well-matured cheese may be a good source. Some people have low levels of folic acid (vitamin B_9) and vitamin B_{12}, which are also important for a normal immune defence system by increasing the effectiveness of the white blood cells. Preferably have the levels of these measured to check that you are not lacking in them.

Support your immune defence forces by supplying them with what they need, training them with physical exercise and winding down stress so that they are not unnecessarily weakened.

Remember!
Strong immune defence is one of the most important weapons in the battle against cancer. Keep your immune defence force strong by keeping it well supplied.

STRATEGY 7:

Every training session counts

W hen I became ill, I didn't have the energy even to think about exercising. It was as if all the strength had been drained from my body. At first, all my energy seemed to be sapped into worrying about the future.

I did remember, however, that exercise had helped me on previous occasions when life was difficult and my mood was low. I had often known grief and sorrow to be dispersed by a good training session. I tried to motivate myself to get going again, but the prospect of better mood was not in itself a sufficient stimulus to tempt me back to the jogging track.

The necessary extra motivation to put my jogging shoes on again came when I discovered recent Danish studies showing what a powerful effect exercise can have in strengthening immune defence and enabling it to combat cancer cells.

I saw that physical activity can help to attack cancer from several directions. Exercise stimulates immune defence, maintains a healthy hormone balance, helps to regulate the blood sugar and also has an anti-inflammatory effect. Regular exercise improves physical health generally and reduces stress.

I have not always been inclined to exercise. As a youngster I was rather sedentary. I preferred reading, using a computer and playing in the band to sweat and effort. However I gradually developed an interest in enjoying the great outdoors, which required me to improve my fitness. It wasn't fun to be always lagging behind the other boys.

In my late teens I decided to apply to officer training school, and from then on there was no turning back; I would need to be fit. I realised that physical exercise gave me energy, self-confidence and a general sense of well-being. My self-image changed gradually, from being the wimp who was always last to be picked for the football team, to seeing myself as good as the next guy.

When the cancer hit me I was glad that I already had experience of exercising to keep fit and knew how to go about it, even though the operations did set me back. Reading about the lethal effects of exercise on cancer cells further increased my motivation.

Physical activity and cancer

Several recent studies show that the incidence of cancer is less among people who are physically active and also that among people who do have cancer, the relapse rate is less in those who are physically active.[43]

Physical activity affects cancer in several ways. Physical training has a direct stimulant effect on the immune system. It is also one of the important influences in maintaining a normal, healthy hormone balance. Physical activity reduces excess levels of oestrogen and testosterone which can stimulate growth of certain cancers (especially in breast, ovary, prostate, uterus and testicle). Exercise also helps to reduce the levels of blood sugar and therefore of insulin and the growth-promoting factor IGF-1. It also reduces the amount of fatty tissue which can absorb and store carcinogenic toxins, and it damps down inflammation, alleviates stress and improves physical health in general.

Other recent research shows how high-intensity training can be particularly beneficial in the battle against cancer. Among other effects, the adrenaline that is secreted into the bloodstream during intense exercise hinders tumours from spreading. As part of the preparation for 'fight or flight,' the high adrenaline levels mobilise the immune system's natural killer cells (NK cells) to find and eliminate the cancer cells.[44]

Another study demonstrated a further enhancement of the effects of exercise. Muscle contraction generated a messenger substance that facilitated the entry of immune cells into cancer tumours.

Even though we know that physical training is good for cancer patients, little has been known about the reason for this. A Danish study has shown that women with breast cancer should do high-intensity training two or three times a week to reduce the risk of spread.[43] The researchers took blood samples from women who were going through a training schedule as part of breast cancer treatment – one specimen before and one after a two hour session of moderate- to high-intensity training. They measured the levels of adrenaline and other substances and also extracted cancer cells from the blood samples. They cultivated these cancer cells in the laboratory for a few days and then implanted them into mice. Among the mice given breast cancer cells from prior to the training session, 90% developed cancer, as compared with 45% of the mice given cells from after the training session. The researchers concluded: 'This indicates that there is something in the blood that restricts the cancer, and that it appears to be related to the adrenaline levels.'[46]

Studies such as this increase our understanding of how physical exercise can hinder the spread not only of breast cancer but of all types of cancer.

How you can do it

I began to think of exercise as a medicine. I used to regard a training session as a sort of happiness pill to blow daily worries and bad moods away with a jog through the countryside, but now I thought of it as an anti-cancer drug where every increase in intensity was an increase in effective dosage. These considerations motivated me to continue training. As I toiled up a hillside during interval training, dripping with sweat, I held in my head a picture of myself receiving treatment through a needle in my arm. I thought of my spurts of intensive exercise as a 'natural' form of chemotherapy, and I re-imagined the picture during each four-minute spurt. Classifying training sessions as a medicine made it easier to motivate myself not to miss a dose. If I wouldn't have missed a dose of an anti-cancer drug, why would I miss a training session?

The pains of physical training seemed to me to be worth the possible benefit, but training doesn't necessarily need to involve pain in the muscles and an unpleasant taste in the mouth. Although studies suggest that more intensive exercise gives greater benefit, what is important is to do *something*. David Servan Schreiber, the author of 'Anti-Cancer,' recommends a half hour of physical activity five times a week. This is in line with official recommendations of physical activity for the population in general. If you do wish to train more intensively, however, you don't need to run as if the devil were at your heels. Interval training at a walking pace can be just as effective for people who may not be in very good form to start with.

Effective interval training

Find a slope that you can walk or run up for a least four minutes at a rapid pace. First, warm up gently for six to ten minutes. Then set off walking quickly up the hill, at a speed that makes you breathless to the extent that it would be difficult to talk. Keep going for four minutes.

Follow this with an 'active pause.' Take four minutes (but no longer) to stroll gently down the hill again.

Leap up the hill again – four minutes.

Repeat the alternating cycle four times.

Then spend six to ten minutes gently winding down. At the

end of this you will have had: six to ten minutes at a gentle pace; sixteen minutes of intensive exercise; twelve minutes between three active pauses; six to ten minutes winding down. You have now done approximately 45 minutes of valuable training!

The interval length of four minutes is not just arbitrary. Research has shown that the heart needs the first two minutes to fill to maximum pump volume. In the last two minutes the heart is working in high gear, with the chambers filled to capacity; that is when you reap maximum benefit. So keep going for four minutes if you can.

If you are already in good form, you will need to run up the slope to achieve the necessary training intensity. If you have a pulse meter, try to keep your pulse rate between 85-90% of your maximum during the high-intensity intervals. You can find your maximum pulse rate either by pushing yourself to the limit or (more easily) by using the rule of thumb and subtracting your age in years from 220. An average 40 year old, for example, would have a maximum recommended pulse rate of about 180 per minute, but individuals vary.

Many people make interval training harder than necessary. It is sufficient to be mildly out of breath, to the extent that would make conversation difficult. You don't need to feel an acrid, metallic taste in your mouth.

On average, maximal oxygen uptake increases by 0.5% with every interval training session.[47] This is good benefit from 45 minutes exercise and much better value than for example from 45 minutes gentle walking on the level. So when you have decided to take advantage of exercise, why not go for maximum benefit?[48]

However, not all exercise needs to be in the form of interval training. It is important for exercise to be varied and enjoyable. Go to the swimming pool, take a bike ride or join in a yoga session. No matter what type of activity you choose, physical exercise stimulates the immune system and makes you more robust.

Are you in too poor shape to exercise just now? If you can

find the energy, know that the greatest benefit comes from the first training session each week. This one session is worth gold. If you can manage two or three spells of exercise that is even better, but you get the greatest benefit from the first. Knowing this makes it easier for many people to find the motivation and the energy to manage at least one session. Having achieved that, you might find a lower threshold to go on to the next one.

Exercise and mental health

In his book Bli hjernesterk ('Strengthen Your Brain'), Swedish doctor Anders Hansen describes how regular physical activity works as well as or better than antidepressant drugs against anxiety and depression.50 Exercise increases the production in the brain of an important substance, known as BDNF ('Brain derived neurotropic factor'). The level of BDNF appears to be low in people who are depressed, and some antidepressant medicines also act by increasing it.

Patience is needed for exercise to have an effect on anxiety and depression. Most people notice a difference after four to six weeks, but it can take six months of regular training to achieve greatest effect.

There are however immediate benefits to be obtained from a training session. Stress level and blood pressure drop immediately and the level of dopamine rises to give a feeling of well-being that can persist for several hours.

Remember!
Every training session counts. Physical exercise works like a medicine to stimulate immune defence, regulate blood sugar and reduce inflammation. Not least, physical activity is also important for psychological health and stress reduction.

STRATEGY 8:

Restrict cancer's capacity to spread

C ould I slow the development of my illness by using every weapon I could find to make life as difficult as possible for the cancer cells? My mission would be a combined operation using all available tactics – every day.

Provided there were promising research results on what I proposed, and provided it was neither harmful nor expensive, what had I to lose by this approach? I had to try. The object-ive had to be to prevent the cancer from spreading further, or at least to restrict it to spreading more slowly. I found research showing that certain foods can slow the spread of cancer.

The route towards my objective was not straightfor-ward, however. First there was a scare along the way.

By autumn 2016 I had come through two operations and a series of subsequent investigations: a PET-CT scan to look for secondary tumours; MRI scans of my head and abdomen; a CT scan of my chest. I felt like a laboratory rat as I went from one in-vestigation to another.

Spending an hour in an MR machine is no fun, but that is nothing as compared with the many long hours spent waiting for results.

One instance made a particular impression on me. I had spent an hour in the MR machine. The radiographer had prob-ably seen from the images that I had tumours in the pancreas. He can't have understood that I knew about these already.

Perhaps my relatively young age gave him a feeling of identification and empathy with me. He laid his hand on my shoulder, looked deep into my eyes and wished me luck. I became anxious and fearful. I took his reaction as a sign that my disease had deteriorated rapidly. I slept but little for several nights thereafter, and the wait for my appointment to discuss the results with the doctor felt very long.

I really felt I was waiting for my death sentence. I was scared. On the one hand, I wanted to have the answer as quickly as possible, and on the other hand I wished that the moment would never come, especially if it was going to cut my life expectancy by forty years.

I expected really bad news when the day finally came. The doctor was very late. Sitting in the waiting room, the conversation between myself and my wife had long since dried up. I was too scared and exhausted to speak. I think Hanne was affected the same way.

The doctor came into the waiting room an hour late. He greeted me warmly, but I sensed that he was keeping something back.

'However, you won't be seeing me today,' he said, 'I've arranged for a senior and more experienced colleague to see you.'

I felt the floor give way under my feet. My heart was in my mouth. We were shown in to the consultant and sat down nervously. The new doctor tried to put us at ease with some small talk, to which I didn't feel able to respond. I was terrified.

Eventually he gave me the opportunity to take the bull by the horns. 'Is there anything in particular you are wondering about?'

'The results of the investigations,' I mumbled.

He came right to the point. 'There appear to be signs of spread.'

I had to accept, then, that my prognosis had worsened. The important thing would be to slow down the disease; I couldn't get rid of it. That was a bitter pill to swallow. Several weeks passed, until suddenly the contradictory message arrived: 'It isn't spreading after all.'

I was immensely relieved. It felt as if I had won an important battle, though I knew that the war wasn't over. The tumours could start spreading at any time.

I wouldn't let it happen! I would throw a spanner in the cancer's works to block its development. I knew already that many patients had achieved promising results in slowing the spread of cancer by the various methods I have described in the previous chapters. I hoped to use these strategies to restrict my own cancer.

I continued looking for additional measures that might be helpful. Recent studies have looked into the effect of various spices. Both fresh and dried forms of basil, turmeric, oregano and rosemary have all shown encouraging results in reducing the growth and spread of an aggressive type of breast cancer.[51]

I was already taking turmeric (along with pepper to increase the absorption). I started sprinkling oregano and rosemary over most of my meals too. I may have overdone it a little, as my meals were no longer edible by anyone with less than an extreme liking for spices.

Cancer spread

In order to thrive, multiply and spread, cancer cells are dependent on their surrounding micro-environment.[52] To compare this with a more familiar local environment, imagine that you are working in an office. Some things need to be correct for you to work comfortably and efficiently. It shouldn't be too warm or too cold, you need electricity for the light and the computer to work, it shouldn't be too noisy, and of course you will want something for lunch.

If all these factors are in place you will probably be able to work efficiently. If the power supply fails and you are cold and hungry it will be difficult to work and you may have you wait until circumstances are more favourable.

The same applies to the micro-environment around the cancer cells. Our various strategies are directed to making this environment hostile to them, to make the cancer cells' mission of metastasising to surrounding tissue and distant organs more difficult. It is estimated that 90% of deaths from cancer are because of metastases.[53]

To succeed in creating metastases (secondary tumours), the cancer cell needs to break loose from the primary tumour, come into the blood or lymphatic circulation, avoid attacks by the immune defence forces and emerge from the circulation to invade a new organ. It then has to start dividing again and establish a new blood supply. To achieve all this, the cancer cell needs to ensure that its immediate environment is suitable for growing new blood vessels.

This micro-environment around cancer cells and tumours is so important that the cancer cells are totally dependent on adjusting it to create a favourable milieu for themselves. To restrict the cancer, we need to hinder this process.

At the same time, we need to see how the cancer cells manage to evade our defence mechanisms. A cell that is not behaving 'normally' should usually die off spontaneously, in response to a message from nearby immune cells telling it to 'commit suicide.' The cancer cells manage to avoid this fate, by producing a substance known as NF-kappa B that makes them less susceptible to the regulating signals. Laboratory research has shown that blocking this substance makes the cancer cells vulnerable again and thereby hinders spread.[54] The growth and spread of cancer is largely dependent on this 'super-weapon.' Without NF-kappa B a cancer cell becomes very vulnerable.

How you can do it

Use herbs and spices that inhibit cancer spread, such as mint, thyme, marjoram, basil, rosemary and turmeric (with pepper).

They work in a similar way to certain types of cancer drugs.[55] The spices are rich in terpene fatty acids which give them their characteristic scent. Terpenes have been shown to work on different types of cancer by reducing spread and enhancing the death of cancer cells. Carnosol, a terpene which is present in rosemary, affects cancer cells' capacity to invade surrounding tissue.

Research has also shown how extracts of rosemary help cytotoxic drugs to penetrate better into cancer cells. Breast cancer cells in laboratory culture appear to have less resistance to cytotoxic drugs if the patient from whom the cells were taken has been given rosemary at the same time.

Eat food that inhibits NF-kappa B.[56] Include these foodstuffs in your daily diet:

Boswellia extract
Capsaicin (in chilli pepper)
Berries
Garlic
Ginger
Green tea
Liquorice root
Omega-3 fatty acids
Oregano
Pomegranate
Resveratrol (in red grapes and red wine)
Turmeric
Vitamin D
Walnuts
Zinc

Examples:
    ½ - 1 teaspoon turmeric with a little black pepper;
    ½ teaspoon root ginger, grated into green tea;
    1 or 2 cloves of garlic (or more) daily, passed through a garlic press;
    (The spices can be either fresh or dried and can be strewn onto

food according to taste.)

Vitamin D; sun or supplements in winter.

Remember!

Preferably combine several of the strategies to restrict spread. Create a hostile environment for the cancer cells. Include herbs and spices such as mint, thyme, marjoram, oregano, basil, rosemary and turmeric in your daily diet. The growth and spread of cancer cells is largely dependent on their production of the inflammation-provoking chemical, NF-kappa B. Choosing foodstuffs that block this will make life more difficult for them.

STRATEGY 9:

Kill cancer cells

A s the various strategies became part of my daily routine, I hoped that my immune defences were becoming capable of dealing with many of the cancer cells. After I had started my self-treatment, I noticed that it was a long time since I had had a cold. Was this just coincidence, or was it a sign that my immune defence had grown stronger? Chemotherapy to kill the cancer cells had not been considered appropriate treatment for me up to now, though I would have accepted it if it had been feasible. I started wondering whether there were 'natural' cytotoxic substances that could exterminate the cancer cells. Again, I found some possible candidates in the plant kingdom.

Some vegetable substances can damage cancer cells. Salvesterols and some other substances in berries, fruit and green vegetables can bring about the death of cancer cells.

If we have cancer we hope that the chemotherapy will work, that the surgeon will manage to remove the whole tumour or that the radiotherapy will melt it away. However, we know that this is not always enough and that some cancer cells may escape.

I wanted to do my utmost to make life difficult for the cancer cells, in addition to the treatment provided by the hospital, and so I now added in daily doses of salvesterols. As I have always been fond of blueberries, eating them was no hardship.

Substances that can help
to kill cancer cells

Several components of food can contribute to the death of cancer cells. In India, where turmeric is in common use, the incidence of lung cancer for example is 1/8 of the incidence in Western countries. The incidence of large bowel cancer is 1/9, breast cancer 1/5 and kidney cancer 1/10 of ours. The difference is even greater for prostate cancer – 1/50. This is despite the population of India often being exposed to just as many carcinogenic toxins as we in the West.[57] Researchers suspect that one of the reasons for this is the widespread use of turmeric, a spice that contains curcumin. This active ingredient induces cancer cells to submit to the programme of cell death.[58]

Other molecules that can work in the same way as curcumin in driving cancer cells to suicide include procyanidins and proanthocyanidins. These are present in various foods, including blueberries, cranberries, cinnamon and dark chocolate. However, blueberries and cranberries are not the only fruits that can be effective against cancer. Animal studies have shown, for example, that black raspberries from Canada have a restraining effect on cancers in the mouth, oesophagus and large bowel in rats. Another trial using powdered raspberry containing large amounts of anthocyanins gave similar results. Both these experiments showed that the rats who ate the berries developed 50% fewer tumours than the rats in the control group.[59] As with other animal studies we should be careful about coming to conclusions about the possibilities for humans, but such results are a significant indication of something that is worth exploring further.

Other substances with exciting possibilities for further investigation are the salvesterols. These 'recognise' cancer cells, penetrate into them and destroy them from the inside, while healthy cells are protected from damage. Salvesterols are attracted to the enzyme CYP_1B_1 which is present in cancer cells but not in healthy cells. Salvesterols are effective straight away: They can kill cancer cells as soon as 30 minutes after ingestion.

How you can do it

As berries can destroy cancer cells, it is a good idea to eat a cupful of berries every day.[60] Always eat organically grown berries.

Fruit and berries that contain salvesterols
Apples
Blackcurrants
Blueberries
Cranberries
Grapes
Mandarins
Strawberries

Vegetables that contain salvesterols
Avocado
Broccoli
Cabbage
Cauliflower
Paprika

Also eat cinnamon and dark chocolate (which contain procyanidins and proanthocyanidins) and also turmeric, to drive the cancer cells to suicide. Half a cup of berries and two or three squares of dark chocolate are suitable amounts per day.

Remember!
The cancer will not thrive if you eat plantstuffs and berries that can help to kill cancer cells. So include foods containing proanthocyanidins, procyanidins and salvesterols as part of your daily diet.

STRATEGY 10:

Cut off the sugar supplies

I once had the unfortunate experience of running out of fuel when driving my car. Suddenly, the tank was empty and the engine refused to fire into life again. I remembered that occasion when I read how dependent cancer cells are on their fuel, glucose. What would happen to them if I cut off their sugar supplies?

I knew that the cancer cells require large amounts of glucose to thrive, grow and spread. So it was sensible to cut down my intake of sugar to make things difficult for them.

The sugar that the cancer cells need in order to grow come from carbohydrates, whether in the form of added sugar or sugars naturally present in foodstuffs such as milk (lactose), fruit (fructose) or beer (maltose). It is important to think about how much carbohydrate you are taking in altogether, so that you can avoid making a big surplus of fuel available to the cancer.

The most extreme method of carbohydrate reduction is a ketogenic diet. This can be difficult to manage. It is not suitable for everybody, though it is a possibility worth considering. However, you can come a long way in cutting down on carbohydrate without going to the full extent of cutting it out completely.

Until recently, I hadn't used a full ketogenic diet. I had

been content to reduce my carbohydrate intake as well as I could, together with using the other strategies I have described.

A ketogenic diet contains very little carbohydrate. It appears to be effective against cancer in several ways. It is probably the most difficult weapon to use, but perhaps also the most effective.

Adam Sorenson in Canada was 13 years old when he was diagnosed with an advanced brain tumour in September 2013. The prognosis was grave; he probably had only a few months to live. The neurosurgeons operated to remove as much of the tumour as possible. As chemotherapy would have had little effect on this type of tumour, he was treated with radiotherapy after the operation. This changed the prognosis only slightly, as his type of tumour was known to be liable to rapid recurrence and further spread.

Adam's parents were desperate and began to wonder whether there were other treatments worth trying. They consulted other doctors and Adam's father started a thorough search of the relevant research reports. Was there anything that could give his son a better chance of survival? He set out criteria that an additional treatment would need to meet:

- It must not be harmful to the boy in any way.
- There must be published clinical research to support it.
- It must be readily available.

A ketogenic diet met all the requirements. The research results were promising, the diet was not harmful and it was readily available – and feasible. Adam did of course find it difficult to forego pizza and other treats, especially when he was with other children, but he understood what his father was trying to do and he managed to stick to the diet, encouraged by the thought that it might help him to survive.

The gloomy prognosis was averted. Adam still attends for regular check-ups, but so far the MRI scans have shown no signs of recurrence of the tumour. He is healthy and leads a normal teenage life, apart from continuing his strict diet. In September 2016, three years after diagnosis, Adam was the keynote speaker at the Global Symposium on Ketogenic Therapies which took place in Alberta, Canada.

Ketogenic diets and cancer

A diet with a reduced content of carbohydrates and calories can help to kill cancer cells, by depriving them of the glucose they need. Cancer cells' 'immortality' largely disappears when the diet restricts the energy available to them. When the energy production from glucose in cancer cells drops, they become liable to cell death and in some instances their growth is stopped. Many researchers refer to cancer's dependence on sugar as its 'Achilles heel.'[61]

What was it that Adam's father had discovered in the scientific literature during his search for hope? Ketones are a product of the metabolism of fats. 'Ketosis' means burning fat rather than sugar. A 'ketogenic' diet based on metabolising fats rather than sugars has been used in the treatment of epilepsy, because it has been shown to reduce the number of seizures. Epilepsy is not usually caused by cancer, though it can sometimes occur when a tumour in the brain causes increased pressure and triggers seizures. Researchers wondered whether a ketogenic diet could restrict the growth of tumours, and further research followed.

Adam's story is one of now many examples of the success of ketogenic diet in controlling cancer. Most of the research on this topic to date has focussed on brain tumours, but the scope is being extended to other forms of cancer. Most studies up to now has been on animals or on cell cultures in laboratories. Many of the animal studies have shown ketogenic diet to be amazingly effective. Among mice who had had brain tumour cells implanted, the tumours melted away in those mice who were given a ketogenic diet. The results of animal studies cannot necessarily be applied to humans, but there are some smaller studies on humans that indicate an effect on brain tumours. Further research is needed to confirm this. There are currently about a dozen clinical studies under way on the effect of ketosis on cancer in humans.

Ketogenic diet can be used as an addition to but not as a substitute for conventional treatment. If you want to follow a ketogenic diet as an ancillary treatment, it is important to work closely with the oncologists so that the overall treatment can be tailored to your particular case as closely as possible.

For many people, 'changing fuel' to a ketogenic diet seems so strange at first glance that it is natural to question whether the body will tolerate it. Our genes have developed under quite different dietary circumstances from those we live in today. Until the agricultural revolution about 13,000 years ago, people had very little access to sugar. Apart from modest amounts of berries and honey, the diet of our distant ancestors consisted mainly of fats, proteins and some plant foods. Our genes developed in adaptation to these circumstances.

So in the absence of sugar our bodies are well capable of burning fat. It is a different story for the cancer cells. They are dependent on large amounts of glucose if they are to thrive, and this dependence makes them vulnerable. You can weaken them by attacking their supply lines.

Most types of cancer depend on glucose to generate energy so that they can multiply and spread. A cancer cell usually has damage in its mitochondrion (its power station) and has to generate energy differently from a normal cell. The cancer cell does this by lactic fermentation, which requires a much bigger supply of glucose than a normal cell uses.

Although the cancer cell faces a disadvantage in needing to acquire so much glucose, it turns this to its own advantage when it gets the chance. When glucose is metabolised to provide energy by this alternative method of lactic fermentation, an excess of carbon becomes available to be used as building material for new cancer cells. The lactic acid that is produced in this process also promotes spread; in an environment rich in lactic acid, it is much easier for the cancer cell to invade surrounding tissue. With a ketogenic diet, you can deny the cancer cell large supplies of glucose.

If you eat very little carbohydrate, your body will switch over to burning fats instead. This releases another type of fuel, known as ketone bodies, that can be metabolised particularly well by healthy cells, but not in general by cancer cells.

Unfortunately, it is not possible to starve the cancer cells to death in this way, as the body ensures that there is always some blood sugar available even if you are eating little carbohydrate. Nevertheless, a ketogenic diet does significantly reduce the tumour's access to sugar.[62] Ketone bodies also suppress inflammation, further restricting cancer spread.

Knowing all this, you can attack four of cancer's weak points:

1. Cut down carbohydrate intake drastically to reduce the supplies available to the cancer cells.
2. Switch your metabolism to fat-burning which produces ketone bodies that the cancer cells cannot use.
3. Ketone bodies normalise the genes within cancer cells.
4. Ketones suppress inflammation.

How you can do it

A ketogenic diet is an extreme variant of a low carbohydrate diet, where the amount of carbohydrate in the diet is kept to a minimum to switch the body over to burning fats. At the same time, protein intake is restricted because much of protein is metabolised to sugar.

The most important thing is to avoid the biggest sources of carbohydrate: bread, pasta, rice, potatoes and so on. To achieve ketosis the total carbohydrate content of the diet needs to be less than 50 grams, possibly as low as 20 grams per day. Also, the intake of protein needs to be restricted to about 1 gram per kilogram of bodyweight per day.

So a person weighing 70 kg. could eat up to 70 grams of protein per day, equivalent to about 250 grams of meat, fish or chicken. A ketogenic diet is particularly rich in fat, not in protein as is sometimes mistakenly thought. A good rule of thumb is to have less than 10% of energy intake from carbohydrates, 15-25% from proteins and 70% or more from fats.

Such diet rich in fat should be avoided for prostate cancer patients and for malignant melanoma, as it seems these types of cancers can readily utilise fats for fuel, unlike most other cancer types.

Ketosis is achieved when the body switches over fully to fat-burning in the absence of carbohydrate in the food. It takes between two and three weeks on a ketogenic diet for this change to happen. Success can be measured by testing the urine with 'Ketostix.'[63]

Note that this diet can conflict with some of the advice I have given earlier. For example, it will be necessary to restrict your intake of nuts and berries (though small amounts are fine).

It is important to stress that this type of diet is not necessarily suitable for everyone. Reducing carbohydrate without going to the extent of inducing ketosis is also an effective weapon.

Remember!

A ketogenic diet makes use of the healthy cells' advantage over the cancer cells; the healthy cells are not so dependent on glucose as the cancer cells. Ketone bodies are a high-grade fuel for the healthy cells. Look into it carefully and preferably discuss it with your oncologist before trying it.

MORE ABOUT
KETOGENIC DIETS

Who should be cautious
about a ketogenic diet?

T hose who struggle to keep their weight up: A ketogenic diet often causes weight loss initially. Discuss it with your doctor.

Those taking drugs for high blood pressure: The blood pressure often drops, and sometimes it drops too far. It is uncertain whether antihypertensive drugs are needed at all when on a ketogenic diet, but the blood pressure should be measured regularly to begin with.

Diabetics on insulin: The insulin requirement often drops dramatically. If the dose is not adjusted accordingly this can lead to potentially dangerous hypoglycaemia (low blood sugar). So close liaison with the doctor or specialist nurse is required.

Diabetics on tablets (especially sulphonylureas). They are also at risk of hypoglycaemia and should consult their doctor.

Women who are pregnant or breast-feeding should not go onto a ketogenic diet.

Some cancer types should avoid high intake of fats: Patients who have prostate cancer and malignant melanoma should be cautious of excess amounts of fats in their diet, discussion with an oncologist should be done before starting a high-fat diet.

Important things to consider before you try it

The metabolism takes at least two weeks to convert to burning fats. The change of diet can cause some discomfort at first. This is transient and not dangerous, and can be alleviated by simple means. The commonest initial problems are slight headache, fatigue, increased thirst and a craving for sweet things. Some people experience leg cramps because of reduced salt intake. These symptoms can be relieved by taking plenty fluids – water with salt and lemon, or bouillon to replace the missing salt.

Some tips

The rule of thumb is to limit the carbohydrate content of your daily diet to less than 20-30 grams and the protein content to 1 gram per kilogram body weight, e.g. 70 g. per day for a person weighing 70 kg.

Eat enough fat to feel satisfied.

Avoid snacking between meals if you aren't hungry.

Examples of carbohydrate and protein content of various foods

Carbohydrate content per 100 grams

Meat	0 gram
Fish and shellfish	0 gram
Eggs	1 gram
Cheese	2 grams
Fats (butter, olive oil, etc.)	0 gram
Green vegetables (not root vegetables)	1-5 grams

Protein content

100 grams of meat, fish or chicken approx. 20 grams	
150 grams chicken fillet	29 grams
20 grams (2 slices) boiled ham	4 grams
20 grams (2 slices) white cheese	5 grams
Small can of mackerel in tomato sauce	15 grams
50 grams cottage cheese	7 grams
One egg	7 grams

What can you eat?

Meat: No restriction. As the ketogenic diet consists of substituting foods rich in fats instead of carbohydrates, you should not discard the fat. If possible select meat that has been grown ecologically, meat from non-domestic animals or meat from animals reared on pasture rather than by artificial feeding.

Fish and shellfish: No restriction. Oily fish such as salmon, brown trout or mackerel are beneficial; preferably wild-caught rather than farmed.

Eggs: In all varieties.

Fats and cooking oils: As the ketogenic diet has a high fat content, it is important to select the right fat or oil. Choose real butter rather than margarine, and always rapeseed oil or olive oil rather than other vegetable oils. Either warm-pressed olive oil or rapeseed oil is suitable for frying, but if you do need to use a cold-pressed olive oil, choose extra virgin olive oil. Palm oil can also be used.

Dairy products: Choose the varieties with high fat content. Real butter and sour cream, fatty cheeses and yogurt (without added sugar). Be sparing with or avoid milk and cream that contains a lot of milk sugar. Cheese is suitable, as it contains a lot of fat and little carbohydrate. Cheese does however contain a certain amount of protein which in large quantities can cause the level of insulin to rise. Cheese should therefore be taken in moderation.

Vegetables

At the beginning:
 Asparagus
 Avocado
 Broccoli
 Brussel sprouts
 Cabbage
 Cauliflower
 Celery
 Cucumber
 Leafy salads
 Mushrooms
 Olives
 Spinach

These can be added when you are in ketosis:
 Garlic
 Onion
 Paprika
Sweet potato
Tomatoes
Berries – These are fine in small quantities, preferably taken with a fat (such as cream without added sugar). Blueberries and raspberries do not raise the blood sugar very much, but strawberries and currants have a bigger effect.
Fruit – To achieve ketosis you will need to limit your intake of fruit. Wait until you are ketotic before re-introducing a little fruit with low sugar content, such as apples or pears,

preferably combining it with some fatty food to restrict the rise in blood sugar.

Nuts – a handful of nuts per day is beneficial, but don't overdo it. If nuts make you feel more hungry, stop eating them. Nuts can cause some people to over-eat.

These types of seeds and nuts are suitable:
Almonds
Brazil nuts
Chia seeds
Hazel nuts
Hemp seeds
Linseed
Macadamia nuts
Pecan nuts (max. 2-3 daily)
Walnuts

Once you have established ketosis, you can also take some peanuts.

Sweeteners – Artificial sweeteners will make you hungrier. Take water, tea or coffee rather than soft drinks. If necessary, however, artificial sweeteners can be a good alternative to sugar. The ones to use are stevia, agave nectar, agave honey or coconut sugar.

Spices – Can be taken safely, but watch out for some spice mixes that can have added sugar or starch.

Drinks – Plain or aerated water (without added tastes)
Tea, preferably green tea
Decaffeinated coffee (Caffeine can raise the blood sugar level.) If you are addicted to coffee, cut down to a small cup after breakfast, or change to decaffeinated coffee.
Coconut milk without added sugar

Almond milk without added sugar

What do you need to avoid on a ketogenic diet?

The most important thing to avoid is sugar: sweets, chocolate, cakes, biscuits, soft drinks, juice.

Chocolate: Can be taken in small quantities, preferably dark chocolate 70% or more. If this stimulates over-eating it should be stopped.

Starches: Bread, pasta, rice, potatoes, chips, crisps, porridge, muesli, breakfast cereals.

Margarine: Choose pure butter instead, because of the unhealthily high content of omega-6 fatty acids in margarines.

Alcohol: Beer contains malt sugars and should be avoided. Dry wine, preferably red, can be taken in small doses, preferably with meals; one glass with a meal so that the sugar in the wine doesn't raise the blood sugar too much. Spirits and other alcoholic drinks should be avoided.

Fruit: Fruit contains a lot of sugar and should be avoided in a ketogenic diet, but can be taken in small quantities if you are implementing the previously described strategies but have decided not to go for a ketogenic diet.

A ketogenic diet is possibly the most difficult of the ten strategies I have described. You can obtain great benefit from applying the other nine without necessarily using the tenth.

Examples of ketogenic meals

Breakfast
Boiled egg
Egg fried in butter or olive oil
Omelette. This can be filled with: spices such as turmeric, pepper, oregano and rosemary; cheese; cabbage; tomato; spring onion; tomato; garlic or other varieties of onion. Sprinkle a little olive oil over the omelette before serving.
Ham, cheese, nuts, vegetables

Lunch
Salads, but without maize or potatoes
Avocado, mozzarella, tomatoes. Sprinkle with olive oil.
Left-overs from yesterday's dinner
Omelette

Dinner
Choose whatever protein source you prefer: meat, fish or chicken. Remember your daily limit for protein intake; 1 gram per kilogram body weight. Use above-ground vegetables rather than root vegetables, which have more sugar and should be avoided at first.
Fats: melted butter, sour cream, olive oil
Drinks: Coffee or tea can have a couple of teaspoons of coconut milk added.

Periodic fasting – an alternative?

Various methods of fasting offer an alternative way to switch the metabolism more rapidly over to burning fat. Periodic fasting can bring about the change quicker and can be useful as a way of starting on a ketogenic diet. Fasting gives many of the same benefits as a ketogenic diet and can be used as an alternative.

Periodic fasting helps to reduce the insulin level, loose weight, suppress inflammation and clean the body of unwanted cellular components ('autophagy').

N.B: Periodic fasting is not suitable for cancer patients who struggle to maintain their weight, for example during chemotherapy when nausea and weight loss are common. People with diabetes (whether on insulin or on tablets) should also consult carefully with their doctor. The same can apply to people on other medicines – always consult your doctor first.

If fasting is suitable for you, try for example the 16:8 method. Fast for 16 hours and eat during the other eight hours. This way you can have a main meal around the middle of the day or during the early afternoon and fast until breakfast the next morning; from 4 p.m. to 8 a.m. would be 16 hours. Alternatively you could have your evening meal slightly later and fast until lunch-time the next day. This can be done once or several times per week.

Another system is the 5:2 method. This consists of eating normally five days per week, followed by two days of fasting during which however you can take in up to 500 kilocalories per day.

Yet another variant is the prolonged fast of 3 to 7 days, which can be used occasionally. This is more demanding and it is advisable to look into it carefully and read as much as you can about it before you start. It is important to maintain your fluid and salt intake. Tea, coffee and clear soup dampen hunger when fasting, but you must also drink plenty water.

Summary

Ten common features of cancer and the strategies for counter-attack.
The signals initiating cell division fail to stop (str. 5, 8)
Avoidance of factors restricting growth   (str. 5)
Avoidance of the immune defences   (str. 3, 5, 6, 7)
Capacity to continue dividing indefinitely   (str. 8)
Inflammation stimulating cancer growth   (str. 4, 5, 7, 8)
Activation of invasion and metastasis   (str. 1, 4, 5, 7, 8)
Creation of new blood vessels   (str. 1)
Mutations   (str. 2)
Avoidance of programmed cell death   (str. 6, 8, 9)
Change in the cancer cell's metabolic processes (str. 10)

Strategy 1: Eat food that damages the cancer cells'
              blood supply.
Strategy 2: Avoid and clear out harmful substances.
Strategy 3: Reduce stress.
Strategy 4: Reduce raised hormone levels and obesity.
Strategy 5: Suppress inflammation.
Strategy 6: Build up your immune defence.
Strategy 7: Physical activity.
Strategy 8: Restrict the capacity to spread.
Strategy 9: Kill cancer cells.
Strategy 10: Reduce the supplies of glucose.

DOES IT WORK?

When I was back in the National Hospital following the second operation, I had been applying these strategies for twelve weeks. I had been eating food that would help me in my battle against cancer, and I had been training regularly. In the hospital I politely declined slices of bread, apple juice and puddings. My dear sister brought me home-made salads to eat instead of the unsuitable hospital food.

The day before my review appointment seemed particularly long. I knew that there were still tumours in my pancreas that couldn't be removed surgically. The big question was whether they had grown. I had been thinking about this inwardly every single day, prompted by fearsome imaginations of the cancer as a wild animal gnawing at my body from inside.

Although I didn't feel any particular symptoms, I kept wondering whether I would recognise signs of the tumour growing or spreading. When you are anxious to know something, one way or the other, it is difficult to know for sure. When the brain is especially alert for symptoms, it detects pains and discomforts more easily. Then fear comes sneaking in, and the brain becomes even more on guard.

'Torp?' the oncologist called into the waiting room.

My pulse rose. My primitive instincts urged me to leave the waiting room and run away, but my legs obeyed higher control and I walked into the consulting room.

I tried to greet the doctor normally and politely, but my stiff, clammy handshake betrayed my fear.

However, there was little reason for fear this time. The images on the screen showed that the tumours had not grown since they were first discovered! I felt enormously relieved, though the oncologist qualified his interpretation: 'This shows that the tumours appear not to be rapidly growing, *but they will undoubtedly grow. Cancer cells multiply; it's in their nature.*'

I heard what he said, but a little voice within me was whispering: 'What if my strategies work and the cancer growth can be stopped after all?'

THE DREAM
BECOMES REALITY

On the day of the Berlin Marathon, a million Berliners and visitors are out in the streets celebrating a gigantic folk-festival in support of the runners. Participants in the race don't get a moment to feel sorry for themselves. Instead, the crowd urges them on to do their best, and a little bit more. The sound of the start signal gives me goosebumps.

There's no way back. The miles lie ahead of me, but it is not the stress of competing that is causing the goosebumps; it's the fact that I really am here. Or to be even more blunt: the fact that I still **am**, still exist. There's not much opportunity to reflect on that in the noise and challenge of the passing miles, but the thought lies smouldering behind it all.

A mass of people lines Torstrasse, and the noise from there hits me as I run over Rosa-Luxembourg-platz. Horn music, laughter and shouts of encouragement blend with the clatter of thousands of feet on the asphalt.

On this September day, 40,000 runners cover 26.2 miles through the streets of Berlin. The course that winds through the town is only slightly hilly and offers the prospect of good times for both professional and amateur runners as we test our bodies right to the finishing line beside the Reichstag Building.

I put the first six miles behind me without difficulty in 45 minutes. I feel fine, running almost automatically. This is what I have been training for. I have wanted to train for it, and I had to train for it. Sixteen miles to the finish, but my goal has already been achieved.

There is joy, relief and success in each step.

I expect to be tired today. I know that Hanne is waiting for me to cheer me on the last few metres to the finish.

26.2 miles.

A year after the operations.

PART 3:

A HANDBOOK OF ANTI-CANCER MEASURES

Food against cancer

E ach of the foodstuffs and other measures that I have suggested has its own effect against cancer, but combining them can give a greater effect than each would have on its own ('synergy'). Their interactions make it a good idea to combine several measures at the same time to attack the cancer on as many fronts as possible.

A complete anti-cancer diet consists of combining various foodstuffs that contain nutrients with powerful anti-cancer properties and that have each individually been shown to have beneficial results. To study the effect against cancer of each nutrient in detail might be an unnecessary diversion, but what matters in the end is the combined effect of all the nutrients acting together. The important thing is what you put on your plate and how well the various foods work together.

There is reason to believe that a diet combining a number of ingredients that are active against cancer in different ways leads to a strong interplay of action against cancer growth. There is no reason to believe that such a diet is harmful to you.

Is it now time for you to start your own cancer project?

TEN STEPS TOWARDS A BETTER PROGNOSIS

I t is often wise to start with the easiest measures first. So I suggest a step by step approach, one step at a time. Even if you do not choose or do not manage to go the whole way, each single step will have an effect and the further you manage to go, the greater the effect you can expect.

First step: drinks and spices

Start by taking nutrients that suppress inflammation and can stimulate your immune system.

Drinks: Green tea, 3 – 5 cups per day

Spices: Add herbs and spices to your food: ½ to 1 teaspoonful of turmeric together with pepper and olive oil. Also season your food with oregano, rosemary, thyme and basil.

See strategies 1, 5 and 7 for further details.

Second step: eat greens

Try to convert your diet gradually towards greens, experimenting and learning as you go. There are many good books and websites to provide inspiration.

See strategy 5 for information, plus the list of the most effective green vegetables.

Third step: 'Vita'(min) means 'life'

Take enough vitamins, especially vitamins C and D that are important for the immune system.
> See strategy 6

Fourth step: Banish sugar

Cancer cells are totally dependent on large supplies of sugar. Don't let them have it!
> Cut down on added sugar and sweets.
> See strategy 10

Fifth step: eliminate toxins

Quit smoking, reduce alcohol use and avoid harmful chemicals. Eat food that helps to clear away toxins.
> See strategy 2

Sixth step: de-stress

Relax! Adapt your lifestyle if necessary. Learn yoga, mindfulness or other relaxation techniques.
> See strategy 3

Seventh step: be physically active

Take regular physical activity of a kind that you enjoy.
> See strategy 7 for the rationale

Eighth step: drop your daily bread

Reduce the carbohydrate content of your diet. Abandon bread, rice, pasta and potatoes. Replace them with other good foods such as omelettes, salads, meat, fish, chicken and nuts. If your craving for bread is too strong, change to low carbohydrate bread or protein bread as an alternative.

Ninth step: periodic fasting

Periodic fasting can be useful to reduce insulin levels, reduce overweight, suppress inflammation and cleanse the body of waste products of cellular metabolism (autophagy).

See strategy 10

Tenth step: ketogenic diet

Try a ketogenic diet so that your healthy cells can use the ketone bodies from metabolism of fats, which cancer cells are unable to do.

See strategy 10

There is no doubt that research is constantly producing more evidence of how you can play a part in improving your chances. Perhaps your lifestyle is such that you are already well on the way with these steps. You don't necessarily need to follow all of them. They are not all suitable for everybody, and there are differences in people's state of health at the start. If you are unsure, ask your oncologist or another appropriate health professional. You don't need to do everything all at once. And remember, every step helps!

What does a day of anti-cancer measures look like?

Breakfast

An omelette is a good base for other healthy foods.

Suggestion: Make a 2-3 egg omelette, cooked in butter or warm-pressed olive oil. Pour the whisked eggs into the pan before turning on the heat. Season with turmeric, pepper, oregano and other spices you choose. Add chopped tomato, garlic, cabbage and whatever cheese you like, plus ham if you wish. The advantage of adding these before you turn on the heat is that the tomatoes will be warmed up gradually in the oil, releasing the carotenoid chemical lycopene, which is a valuable anti-oxidant. Some researchers also advise that it is advantageous for the turmeric to be warmed up in the oil in the same way.

Sprinkle a little olive oil over the omelette when it is ready, and sprinkle some nuts on top. You will feel satisfied for a long time, and your blood sugar will remain stable for several hours.

Drink: green tea, preferably with grated root ginger.

Lunch

Benefit from the health-giving properties of the plant kingdom. Make up a salad from the list of the green vegetables that are most effective. Sprinkle olive oil on it, and supplement it with tuna fish, cheese or ham if you wish. I often add spices too.

Drink: Green tea.

Dinner

Fish, meat or chicken. Wild-caught rather than farmed fish if possible, and free-range rather than domestically reared meat or chicken. All with a generous accompaniment of vegetables.

Drink: water, mineral water or tea

Dessert? A bowl of berries. Frozen berries are just as effective as fresh berries.

Late evening

I don't always feel the need for a late evening snack, but sometimes I eat left-overs from dinner or a few nuts, some vegetables or a little cheese or ham.

Drink: Green tea

If you have managed to include a training session in the course of the day you will have applied most of the ten recommended strategies!

Old habits die hard.

Changing established habits is challenging. Food is an important part of our lives, a source both of pleasure and of anxiety. Eating habits are learnt young and are very persistent. It can appear impossible at first glance to change such an ingrained habit. Many people have tried various slimming regimens to lose weight and seen their weight fall, only to creep up again when they stop the diet.

If you want to change a habit, it is important to change to something that suits you even better than your previous way. You may not miss your previous diet once you have made the change; many find their new diet even tastier and more attractive than their old one. Changing from a traditional diet rich in bread and carbohydrate to a diet based more on vegetables and pure natural ingredients such as meat, fish and chicken gives more and richer flavour.

People often point out to me that such a diet is expensive. Pure basic ingredients of meat, fish, chicken, cheese, eggs and vegetables are often more expensive than a wider diet, but look at the broader picture; you may have stopped smoking and given up chocolate, sweets, sweet drinks and other things. Anyway, most of us agree that it is worthwhile to invest in our own health.

A new routine

A meal consisting of anti-cancer foods may look different from what you are accustomed to. Many people already know of 'the plate model for healthy eating' as recommended by health authorities. Roughly speaking, this says that you should fill your plate 1/3 with protein foods (meat, fish, eggs), 1/3 with carbohydrate (potatoes, pasta, rice) and 1/3 with salads or vegetables.

An anti-cancer plateful on the other hand is mainly greens, preferably dressed with a healthy oil such as olive, rapeseed or linseed; plus garlic, nuts, herbs and spices. A smaller proportion of the plate holds fish, meat, chicken or egg.

Drink water or tea with your meals. It is good to vary the vegetables, but preferably choose those recognised as particularly capable allies in combatting cancer. Most desserts are best avoided, but take a dish of nature's sweet cancer-suppressing wonder-workers – berries. You can also add in a few squares of dark chocolate (minimum 70%) that are full of antioxidants.

Components of an anti-cancer diet

Olives and olive oil (See strategies 3 and 5)

Olive oil is rich in anti-oxidants (phenols). These can help to inhibit the first phase of cancer development and can reduce the risk of cancers of the breast, bowel and uterus.[64] Black olives are richer in anti-oxidants than green olives. Select cold-pressed, extra-virgin olive oil to pour on as a dressing. A warm-pressed olive oil is better for frying, because it reaches higher temperatures. Olive oil is a good source of healthy lipids. Also, sprinkling olive oil over a salad will make you feel satisfied for longer.

Green tea (See strategies 1 and 3)

Because of its numerous beneficial effects, this amazing drink has already been mentioned several times. Green tea is used throughout the world, and its effects have been widely researched.

In animal studies, researchers have discovered that green tea blocks the effects of harmful chemicals associated with cancer of the breast, lung, oesophagus, stomach and large bowel.

Green tea has also been shown to restrict the growth of tumours in the skin, lung, liver, stomach, breast and large bowel. The tea plant is rich in a type of polyphenol known as catechins. One of these substances has been shown to be particularly effective in blocking the development of new blood vessels. Another substance present in green tea, epigallocatechin (EGCC) hinders the growth of cancer cells in several ways.[65] It stimulates liver enzymes that inactivate carcinogenic substances, and it promotes the natural process of cell death in cancer cells. Green tea also enhances the action of radiotherapy.

Other studies have shown that between three and five cups of green tea per day can reduce the growth of cancer cells.[66] Note that the tea must simmer for at least five and preferably ten minutes to be able to release the active catechins.

Two researchers who studied the relationship between tea drinking and ovarian cancer among 61,057 women over a period of three years found that women who drank at least one cup of green tea per day reduced their risk of death from ovarian cancer by 56 per cent.[68]

A study from Harvard between 1998 and 2009 showed a relationship between consumption of green tea (at least three cups per day) and a reduced risk of recurrence of breast cancer.[69] A bigger study in Japan demonstrated a relationship between tea-drinking and advanced prostate cancer in men.[70]

Herbs and spices (See strategy 8 and 9)

Use herbs generously. Herbs such as mint, thyme, marjoram, oregano, basil and rosemary can be taken every day. These are rich in terpene fatty acids, that give them their characteristic scent. Terpenes help to inhibit cancer from spreading and induce cancer cells to die. For example, a terpene called carnosol which is present in rosemary counteracts the capacity of cancer cells to invade neighbouring tissue. Research has also shown how extracts from rosemary enhance the entry of cytotoxic drugs into cancer cells.[71] Breast cancer cells grown in laboratory culture appear to have less resistance to cytotoxic substances if extract of rosemary is applied at the same time.

Thyme, basil, tarragon, rosemary and oregano are the herbs with the highest content of antioxidants that enable them to attack cancer cells and protect healthy cells. Oregano tops the league, with 138 mmol of antioxidants per 100 grams dry weight. Anything over 75 mmol per 100 grams is considered very high. One gram of dried oregano contains as much antioxidants as the average person ingests in fruit every day.

Antioxidants in herbs:

Oregano:	138 mmol per 100 grams dried weight
Salvia:	90 mmol
Mint:	75 mmol
Lemon balm:	75 mmol
Thyme:	70 mmol
Basil:	30 mmol
Coriander:	3.5 mmol
Parsley:	3.5 mmol

Turmeric (See strategies 1 and 5)

Turmeric is a plant of the ginger family. The root of the plant is what gives the curry powder its yellow colour. Curcumin, one of the substances present in the plant, is one of the most powerful natural anti-inflammatory agents known. In laboratory experiments, curcumin has been shown to suppress the growth of many types of cancer including leukaemia and cancers of the large bowel, lung, liver, stomach, breast and ovary. Curcumin blocks the creation of new blood vessels (angiogenesis) and renders cancer cells susceptible to programmed cell death (apoptosis). It can also protect normal cells from collateral damage by chemotherapy or radiotherapy, and it has been shown to be an effective suppressant of NF-kappa B.[72]

In India, where turmeric is widely used, the incidence of lung cancer for example is 1/8 of the incidence in western countries. The ratios for other cancers are comparable: large bowel 1/9; breast 1/5; kidney 1/10 and prostate 1/50. This is even though the exposure to potentially carcinogenic agents is as great in India as it is in the West.[73]

N.B: for turmeric to be absorbed effectively it needs to be taken along with pepper. Piperin, a substance present in pepper, increases the absorption of turmeric by 2,000 per cent.

Half a teaspoonful of turmeric daily, taken with a little pepper, is a sufficient dose, especially if taken with olive oil too, as this also enhances uptake. Turmeric can be mixed into salads, soups, and dressings, added to tea or sprinkled on omelettes or other dishes.

Ginger (See strategies 1 and 5)

Like turmeric, ginger contains effective anti-inflammatory substances and inhibits the formation of new blood vessels. It also increases the absorption of turmeric. A cup of green tea with added turmeric and a teaspoonful of grated ginger root can be a good way to achieve a combined effect. Ginger can also be added to salads, stir-fries and dressings.

Nuts, berries and fruit (See strategies 1 and 3)

Many berries and nuts contain ellagic acid, a polyphenol which is a very effective detoxicant. It acts by combining certain toxic substances into harmless compounds Ellagic acid is present in raspberries, blueberries, cloudberries and strawberries.

Nuts in the diet can reduce inflammation and reduce the incidence of damage to DNA within cells. They are also a good source of polyunsaturated fats, protein, fibre, vitamin E, magnesium, potassium and antioxidants.

Berries are powerful inhibitors of new blood vessel formation. Cherries are also good detoxicants, because they contain glucuronic acid, which is also present in hazel nuts and walnuts. Rose hips, crowberries, blueberries, black currants, morello cherries, blackberries, raspberries, cloudberries, strawberries, lingonberries and black chokeberries all appear to be very effective against unrestrained cell division.[74]

Salvesterols are phytochemicals present in various berries and plants. They 'recognise' cancer cells, penetrate into them and destroy them. Normal cells are protected against this damage. Salvesterols recognise an enzyme, CYP1B1, which is found in cancer cells but not in healthy cells.

Salvesterols work fast. They can kill cancer cells within 30 minutes after ingestion. Salvesterols can be obtained from the following fruits and berries (preferably grown organically):

Apples
Black currants
Blueberries
Cranberries
Grapes
Mandarins
Strawberries

Citrus fruits such as oranges, grapefruit and lemons contain flavonoids that can suppress inflammation and stimulate detoxification of carcinogenic substances in the liver.

Researchers in one study found that flavonoids (tangeritin and nobiletin) from mandarin peel promoted natural cell death in brain cancer cells.[75] Sprinkle grated citrus fruit peel (preferably organically grown to avoid chemical sprays) in salad dressings or take it in warm water with tea.

Pomegranate juice has been used as a medicine since ancient times and is known to be a powerful antioxidant. In one study, a daily dose of pomegranate juice was shown to reduce the rate of cancer spread by 67 percent.[76] The recommended daily amount is one glass of pomegranate juice. Nectarines, plums and other stoned fruits have also shown good results. One plum contains as much antioxidant substances as a handful of berries, for example.

Eat a cupful of berries daily. Remember that coffee especially can block the absorption of vitamins. So don't drink coffee with the berries. A handful of nuts every day is also beneficial.

Vegetables (See strategy 8)

Cabbage (Brussels sprouts, Chinese cabbage, broccoli, cauliflower) contains sulforaphane and indole-3 carbinols (I_3c). One study showed that this contributed to inhibiting cell division in breast cancer cells.[77] Among other effects, the antioxidant sulforaphane appears to be able to stimulate the immune system's NK cells to act against cancer cells. In an animal study, mice that were given sulforaphane in their diet had half the risk of cancer spread as compared with mice who were not given sulforaphane.[78]

Carrots and beetroot have been shown to be able to inhibit the growth of various types of cancer, including certain gliomas (brain tumours). Beta carotene from these vegetables is absorbed best when they are warmed. Olive oil further increases the uptake. All richly coloured vegetables – red, orange, yellow or green – contain vitamin A and lycopene; tomatoes, paprika or chilli, for example.

Dark green vegetables and avocado contain green lutein. Lutein, lycopene, and canthaxanthin stimulate the immune system and make it more effective. Lycopene in tomato is released when the tomatoes are warmed, either by boiling or by frying lightly in a little oil, which will further increase the absorption.

Onions contain phytochemicals that are also effective against cancer. Garlic has a long history of medicinal use, recorded as early as 3,000 B.C. During World War ll, garlic was called 'Russian penicillin' because of its bactericidal properties and was important when the antibiotic was in short supply. Garlic appears to promote programmed cell death in several types of cancer. Its active molecules are released when the garlic is shredded and are absorbed more easily if a little oil is added.

Garlic also regulates the blood sugar. This reduces production of insulin and IGF-1, thereby reducing cancer cell growth.

Just like berries, several vegetables contain salvestrols that can kill cancer cells. These include:

Avocado
Broccoli
Cabbage
Cauliflower
Paprika

Combine the vegetables to benefit from effective interactions (synergy) in your own body. If you eat several vegetables in one meal, their beneficial effects can enhance each other. An animal study gave interesting results in this context. Rats with prostate cancer were given a combination of broccoli and tomatoes in quantities corresponding to a normal diet in humans. In rats given the combination, the tumours shrank by 52 percent on average, as compared with 32 percent in the rats given only tomato or 42 percent in those given only broccoli. Among rats given only lycopene (a cancer-inhibiting substance in tomatoes), the tumours didn't shrink by more than 18 percent.[79] Tomatoes contain several other active substances in addition to lycopene: vitamins C, E and K; dietary fibre; folic acid; polyphenols and carotenoids.

Pulses (See strategy 8)

Peas, beans and lentils are the edible seeds of leguminous, pod-bearing plants. Their high content of protein and fibre and relatively low carbohydrate content means that they do not cause significant rises in blood sugar levels. They are also high in vitamins, minerals and antioxidants. Beans contain iron, calcium, potassium, selenium, zinc, folic acid and several other B vitamins. Note that 'peanuts' are also a pulse, and not really a nut as many suppose. A metanalysis in 2017 concluded that pulses have a protective effect against prostate cancer.[80] In laboratory studies, substances found in pulses appear to restrict the division of cancer cells and retard tumour growth.[81]

Fish and seafood (See strategy 7)

The harvest of the sea includes nutrients that protect against cancer, such as selenium, vitamin D, vitamin B_{12} and omega-3 fatty acids, all of which strengthen the immune system. The omega-3 fatty acids DHA and EPA also have anti-inflammatory properties. Studies have shown a significant reduction in the risk of several types of cancer in people who eat fish at least twice a week.

Mushrooms (See strategy 6)

Several species of mushroom can stimulate the immune system.

Japanese mushrooms such as shiitake, maitake, kawaratake and enokitake contain a molecule called lentinan. This and other substances present in these mushrooms stimulate the immune system directly.

In Japan, the incidence of stomach cancer is 50% lower in people who eat large quantities of these mushrooms as compared with people who do not.[82] Studies at the Japanese University Hospitals showed a rise in both the number and the activity of immune cells in patients given mushroom extracts.[83]

Another substance present in these mushrooms is AHCC (active hexose correlated compound). This is also available in capsule form as a dietary supplement. It increases the production of important immune cells. It is used in hospitals and clinics in Asia and it is also known to reduce the side-effects of chemotherapy.[84] Many of the types of mushrooms that can be effective against cancer are also obtainable in western countries. Many mushrooms are full of protective antioxidants.

Chaga (*Inonotus obliquus*) is a fungus that grows on birch trees. It has been used by indigenous populations throughout the Northern Hemisphere and is recognised in folk medicine as a treatment for a variety of ailments. Chaga extract can be bought from health food companies. A study on mice in 2016 gave promising results. Chaga was associated with a 60% reduction in tumour size and a 25% reduction in metastases.[85]

An Australian study in 2009 showed that Chinese women who ate 10 grams of fresh mushroom and 4 grams of dried mushroom daily reduced their risk of developing breast cancer by 64%. If they combined this with drinking green tea, the risk fell by as much as 89%.

Portobello mushrooms have also been shown to be effective against cancer. This type of mushroom contains various B vitamins and a number of minerals.

Maitake mushrooms have recognised anti-cancer properties. Several studies have shown that extracts from maitake mushrooms can stop the growth of tumours and strengthen the immune defences in mice with cancer. Maitake can also be effective in the treatment of leukaemia, stomach cancer and bone cancer.

Shiitake has also been shown to be effective against cancer, and **oyster mushrooms** have been shown experimentally to be effective against breast cancer cells and bowel cancer cells.

Reishi is probably the world's most widely used medicinal mushroom. In Japan it is known as the 'phantom mushroom,' because it is so difficult to find. Reishi has for centuries been one of the most highly esteemed immune-strengthening agents in oriental medicine. Taoists call it 'the mushroom of immortality,' and once upon a time it was only eaten by royalty. In Japan, the use of reishi is regarded as a well-tried treatment for some types of cancer and it has been used safely and to good effect, often in combination with other drugs and radiotherapy. It has also been documented as helping to reduce the side-effects of various chemotherapy drugs and radiotherapy.[87]

Red wine (See strategy 1)

Red wine contains resveratrol, a polyphenol that can reduce the activity of NF-kappa B. Resveratrol also blocks the formation of new blood vessels that is so important for the survival of a cancerous tumour. A quantity of not more than one glass of red wine daily is recommended, preferably a dry wine (less than 5 grams sugar per litre) and taken with food to avoid a surge in the blood sugar level.

Dark chocolate (See strategy 1)

The darker the chocolate, the better; preferably more than 70%. Dark chocolate contains antioxidants, plus substances including polyphenols and proanthocyanidins that have the potential to inhibit the formation of new blood vessels and restrict tumour growth.

However, we must remember that chocolate contains sugar and the amount should be limited to a couple of squares per day.

Omega-3 fatty acids (See strategy 5)

Omega-3 fatty acids found in fish and fish oils have been shown to suppress inflammation. DHA (docosahexaenoic acid) and EPA (eicosapentaenoic acid) appear to be the most beneficial. Laboratory research has shown that omega-3 fatty acids reduce the growth of various types of cancer cells (lung, breast, bowel, prostate and kidney).

Omega-3 fatty acids have not been proven to slow cancer cell growth or increase survival in patients with the disease, but they have been shown to improve quality of life because they improve appetite. Taking omega-3 fatty acids can improve the effectiveness of chemotherapy and radiotherapy.[88] They are found not only in fish but also in flax seed, linseed oil, rapeseed oil and olive oil.

Selenium (See strategy 6)

Selenium is an element that is plentiful in organically grown fruit and vegetables and in fish and shellfish. Modern methods of agriculture have led to a drastic fall in the amount of selenium in foodstuffs in recent decades.[89] Selenium appears to stimulate the immune cells (particularly the NK cells) to kill cancer cells more effectively.[90] It is also a powerful antioxidant. Total daily intake should not exceed 400 micrograms. Brazil nuts are a good source of selenium.

Evening primrose oil (See strategy 5)

Oil is extracted from the fruits of the evening primrose plant (*Oenothera biennis*), where it is present in large quantity in the seeds. This plant originated from North and South America, but it has now spread throughout Europe and into parts of Asia.

The roots, stalks, leaves and flower buds of evening primrose are all edible. When boiled, the roots develop a nutty flavour reminiscent of parsnip. The plant can be used in soups and stews, and the young leaves added to salads or boiled as a vegetable. The flowers are also edible. Unripe seed-heads can be boiled or stir-fried.

Since ancient times, the stalk and the leaves have been used to extract oils or the leaves have been applied to relieve inflammation and dress minor wounds. Liquid from boiled leaves has also been used internally for sore throats and digestive problems. More recently, evening primrose oil has mostly been used in the treatment of conditions characterised by chronic inflammation, such as atopic eczema and arthritis.[91]

In laboratory tests, the fatty acid GLA (gamma-linoleic acid) that is present in evening primrose oil led to the death of cancer cells by apoptosis, suppression of new blood vessel formation and enhancement of the effects of radiotherapy and chemotherapy.[92] Laboratory investigations have also shown that GLA is effective against more than forty different types of cancer. One study where operators painted GLA onto brain tumours and surrounding tissue during brain surgery showed signs of the tumours becoming smaller and patient survival rates better.[93]

Patients on some types of antipsychotic drug (e.g. perphenazine) should speak to their doctor before starting evening primrose oil. Also, as evening primrose oil can affect the action of anaesthetic drugs, it should be stopped two weeks prior to a surgical operation.

Coenzyme Q10 (Ubiquinone) (See strategy 6)

In the 1960s, researchers observed that cancer patients often had low blood levels of coenzyme Q10, which was thought to stimulate the immune system and work as an antioxidant. A small study led by Karl Folkers reported that disease progress was slowed in patients taking coenzyme Q10.[94] Several studies support this finding, though it has not yet been fully documented. One study in 2017 concluded that coenzyme Q10 can be effective against a particular type of liver cancer (hepatocellular cancer).[95]

Soya (See strategies 1 and 4)

There is debate about whether soya is effective against cancer or whether, on the contrary, it carries increased risk. Soya contains substances similar to oestrogens, the female sex hormones, and there is some concern that taking soya might be hazardous for people with breast cancer. Many women with breast cancer have therefore been advised to restrict their intake of soya, though the American Cancer Society says that such advice is groundless. Even though the isoflavones in soya can have a slight oestrogenic effect, they also have anti-oestrogenic properties. A big study in China showed that women who had eaten soya throughout their whole adult life had a lower risk of breast cancer.[96]

Studies on men who had had prostate cancer showed that in men who ate soya the PSA (prostate specific antigen) level in blood tests could fall, indicating a reduction in tumour activity. The level fell more slowly in men with active cancer. Like green tea, soya restricts the formation of new blood vessels.

Fibre?

Many people recommend a high fibre diet for good health. High fibre foods such as legumes, whole grain products, fruit, berries and vegetables probably give some protection against cancer.[97]

Fruit is a good example of how fibre can be beneficial. Fruit can contain large quantities of sugar (fructose), but the fibre content will prevent rapid absorption of the sugar and help to stabilise the blood sugar level. Note, however, that you will not get this benefit from drinking fruit juice, which lacks fibre and can therefore lead to rapid rises in blood sugar.

Fat

There is an old myth that eating fat will automatically cause us to put on weight. This will happen if we eat large quantities of fat, because fat is the nutrient with the highest calorie content per gram. In practice, however, our appetite is soon satisfied when we eat food rich in fat and our intake becomes self-limiting.

Also, we feel satisfied for longer when we have eaten food high in fat. This is because fat doesn't increase insulin secretion significantly, the blood sugar level remains stable and the hunger signals that urge us to eat again are not triggered. Try the experiment for yourself, to see how soon you feel hungry after a carbohydrate meal as compared with a fatty meal.

Authorities disagree about whether fat is dangerous. Our fear of fat appears to have been exaggerated, and recent official dietary advice is open to having more fat in the diet again.[98]

What has emerged in recent years is that fat alone cannot be blamed for cardiovascular diseases. Sugar must also be held responsible to some extent. While the experts argue the case, you can choose healthy fats with a good conscience, meantime keeping your insulin and blood sugar levels normal. Preferably choose fats from fish and from olive oil, coconut palm oil, rapeseed oil, avocado, nuts, etc.

Some tips

I use genuine butter, preferably blended with rapeseed oil or olive oil.

I am not scared to eat fat, but I try to avoid meat from animals that have been fed artificially as that can lead to an imbalance between omega-3 and omega-6 fatty acids. You should have as much as possible of the former, but too much of the latter can promote inflammation and be damaging to health.

The ratio of omega-3 to omega-6 fatty acids should preferably be as near 1:1 as possible. In many western countries the average diet contains more omega-6 than omega-3, an unhealthy imbalance.

Which vegetables should you choose?

It's good to vary and mix vegetables. One vegetable may contain substances that are beneficial in a particular way, another may be beneficial in a different way and together they may complement each other.[99]

The vegetables that have shown the most promise against bowel cancer:

Asparagus
Aubergine
Broccoli
Brussels sprouts
Carrots
Cauliflower
Celery
Cos lettuce
Cucumber
Endives/chicory
Fennel
Fern shoots
Garlic

Green beans
Kale
Leek
Onion
Pak Choy
Potatoes
Radish
Red beetroot
Red kale
Red paprika
Shallots
Spinach
Squash
Tomatoes
Turnip

The Top Ten Vegetables

It's a good idea to eat vegetables, and even better to choose the most effective ones.[100] Here are the vegetables most effective in my opinion, ranked from 1 to 10:

1. Garlic, shallots, onions, leeks
2. Brussels sprouts, kale, green kale, Savoy kale
3. Cauliflower
4. Broccoli
5. Red beetroot
6. Spinach
7. Asparagus
8. Bracken shoots
9. Celery
10. Turnip

How much sugar is there in your food?

The most important thing is not to feed the tumour with sugar. So you need to be aware how much sugar there is in various foods. As a sugar lump corresponds to approximately 2 grams of carbohydrate, you can reckon as follows:

> Wholemeal barley bread: One slice equals about 11 sugar lumps
> Oatmeal bread: One slice equals about 6 sugar lumps
> Wheat bread: One slice equals about 6 sugar lumps
> Soft white bread: One slice equals about 7 sugar lumps
> Dark bread: One slice equals about 6 sugar lumps
> Pitta bread: One slice equals about 6 sugar lumps
> Rye bread: One slice equals about 8 sugar lumps
> Apple (120 g.): One apple equals about 4 sugar lumps
> Banana (120 g.): One banana equals about 10 sugar lumps
> Basmati rice(150g.): One portion equals about 20 sugar lumps
> Broccoli (80 g.): One portion equals about 0.4 sugar lumps
> Egg (60 g.): One egg is equivalent to 0 sugar lumps
> Frozen peas: One portion equals about 2.5 sugar lumps
> Maize (80 g.): One portion equals about 8 sugar lumps
> Potato chips (150 g.): One portion equals about 15 sugar lumps
> Potatoes (150 g.): One portion equals about 18 sugar lumps
> Spaghetti (180 g.): One portion equals about 13 sugar lumps

Alcohol

Alcohol is full of carbohydrates. Beer is like rapid-action bread. The phrase 'beer belly' is not without foundation. The maltose sugar in beer causes a rapid rise in blood sugar levels. For example, 500 ml. of pilsner contains 16 grams of carbohydrate, mostly in the form of maltose, equivalent to 8 sugar lumps. The energy from alcohol breakdown must be added . A glass of champagne will give you 1 gram of carbohydrate, and a glass of dry red wine will give you about 2 grams. 'Light' beers contain about 5 grams of carbohydrate per 500 ml. and are therefore a better choice than stronger beers.

Physical Activity

Suggested training programmes

Here are some suggested training programmes. It's not a failure if you can't follow the whole programme. If you can manage one session a week, that's fine, but it isn't essential to follow a strict programme every week. Look on training as a health bonus, and remember that every training session makes a difference.

The hiker

Take a half-hour walk five times a week. Try to make your pulse rate rise a little, and try to walk over varied terrain.

The cyclist

Cycle for 30 – 40 minutes, either outdoors or indoors on an exercise bike, five times a week. Perhaps combine this with a shopping trip or your journey to work or other activity of daily life.

The all-rounder

Combine walking, cycling, swimming or other exercise for half an hour, five times a week.

The enthusiast I

Day 1: Interval hill training. Warm up 6-10 minutes. Walk up and down the slope for four minutes, four times with 3-4 minutes active pause.
Day 2: Rest.
Day 3: Walk, cycle or run at your usual pace, 30 minutes.
Day 4: Rest.

Day 6: Rest.
Day 7: Walk, cycle or run at your usual pace, 30 minutes.

The enthusiast II

Day 1: Interval hill training. Warm up 6-10 minutes. Walk up and down the slope for four minutes, four times with 3-4 minutes active pause.
Day 2: Rest.
Day 3: Strength training at home: Warm up by walking or cycling. Try to do the strengthening exercises four times with a short pause between each session. Any of the following exercises is suitable, repeated a suitable number of times (say 10 – 20) each time:

> Knee squats, under own bodyweight;
> Lunges, under own bodyweight;
> Sit-ups;
> Push-ups;
> Hang-ups;
> etc.

If you go to a gym to train, you can benefit from an instructor's advice.
Day 4: Rest.
Day 5: Interval hill training. Warm up 6-10 minutes. Walk up and down the slope for four minutes, four times with 3-4 minutes active pause.
Day 6: Rest.
Day 7: Strength training.

Ball games

When you are playing, you don't feel tired so quickly. Anyone for tennis, squash, football or golf, for example?

Relaxation

Relaxation exercises can help you to 'unwind' both physically and mentally, easing both physical and psychological tension. A short session of yoga, meditation or breathing exercises can do much to reduce stress and induce calm. The effect is measurable; just count your resting pulse rate or measure your blood pressure for objective evidence of the benefit.

Yoga

Yoga can be very effective in reducing stress, by a combination of physical and mental techniques that include controlled breathing, meditation and physical exercise. Yoga is often useful in helping to control anxiety and relieve psychological distress.

Bodily self-awareness and active breathing enhance relaxation, concentration and energy levels, with additional physical benefits in suppleness strength and balance.[101]

'MediYoga' is a variety of yoga specially developed for therapeutic use. It is physically and psychologically less demanding but makes good use of breathing techniques and meditation. Some hospitals offer MediYoga as part of the treatment for chronic pain and in rehabilitation after cancer treatment. Regular MediYoga sessions have been shown to improve sleep, reduce anxiety and increase confidence and a sense of well-being.[102]

Mindfulness

Mindfulness is the use of simple, practical techniques to train oneself to be fully aware in the here and now. By concentrating on what is happening in your body and mind, you can dispel harmful stress, concentrate your energy and learn to be aware of your thoughts and feelings rather than being controlled by them.

Mindfulness exercises invite you to observe gently what is in your mind from moment to moment, in order to give you an ordered perspective on your thoughts, feelings and bodily sensations, recognising them as part of human nature. You practise accommodating unpleasant thoughts, feelings and sensations without automatically reacting to them.

Mindfulness exercises have been widely used in the treatment of anxiety, stress and depression, because these conditions entail subconscious and sometimes automatic mechanisms to control or avoid unpleasant emotions. Mindfulness training is an attempt to provide yourself with more conscious and flexible responses to yourself and to others.[103]

Practising mindfulness and self-awareness can help us in facing pain and suffering.[104]

Mental strategies

Coping with worrying thoughts

It is difficult not to be frightened when your life is threatened. Fear and worry are natural reactions, but they are also pervasive and tiring. They lead to stress, and chronic stress is not helpful either generally or to somebody who has been stricken with cancer.

Mental strategies are helpful in ridding yourself of anxiety and thereby reducing chronic stress. Cognitive therapy, for example, can help people troubled by worrying thoughts, by enabling them to be more consciously aware of their thought processes and to prevent their anxieties from sapping energy and causing pain.

People who are seriously ill may have many difficult thoughts running through their heads. It is important to focus these thoughts not on what can be lost as a result of the illness but on whatever is good about life.

It makes a big difference to you whether you consider

your glass half-full or half-empty.

Example

John has learned that he has cancer. His thoughts centre on everything he has lost, all the future years that he may never see. Will he become a mere shadow of himself, a weak, sick person who is more of a burden than a help to others? How can he afford to live if he is unable to work? Will his family cope or will his illness ruin things for all of them?

Such damaging thoughts are not at all helpful to John. The more he thinks like that, the more frightened and disheartened he becomes. A vicious circle of negative thoughts and feelings develops, takes control of his life and pulls him further down.

A counsellor helps John to try to change the way he responds to the situation. John comes to understand that he cannot choose what thoughts come into his head, but that he *can* choose how he responds to them. Are these catastrophic preoccupations useful? Are they worth wasting time on? Or will he just accept that they are there but not expend time and energy on them?

Passing clouds

Thoughts come uninvited, but you can let them pass away.

Think of your worries as clouds in the sky. Do you have to grab them and pull them down over your head so that you are enshrouded in grey and mist? Or can you choose to acknowledge that they are there, and then let them float away without giving them further thought?

John realises that it is important to practise dealing with his forebodings. Thoughts are not reality; they are only ideas, and a repeated thought is no more a reality than a transient one. There is a choice to be made which thoughts are worthy of time and attention and which are not.

Many people are unaware that they can make this choice. Try it out, one worry at a time. Are they worth an expenditure of time and energy?

Imagine that you are standing at a railway station and that your worries are like an approaching train. You can choose to get on the train and accompany your worries on the journey, or you can opt to remain standing on the platform and see your worries disappear over the horizon.

This method of handling your worries cannot be mastered without practice, but it is worth an investment of time and effort.

Don't chase pink elephants

Note that John's counsellor didn't ask him to suppress his negative thoughts or cultivate unrealistically positive ones, which can often have the counter-productive effect of making the pain worse.

Trying really hard to suppress a thought can have the opposite effect; the thought just commands more attention. Try NOT thinking about a PINK ELEPHANT. Can you do it? The more you try, the stronger becomes your mental image of the pink elephant. The thought is floating free and will not be stopped.

However, you do have the capacity to influence how much attention to pay to the thought, how much you will believe it and how it will affect you.

The worry hour

The counsellor recommended that John should be allowed to brood over the difficult issues he was facing – but only on Wednesdays from 6 to 7 p.m. He could fret over them as much as he wanted during that hour, but during the rest of the week his negative thoughts should be booked into the worry hour on Wednesday.

Count your blessings

The counsellor asked John to write a list of all the things he was enjoying in life, despite his illness. He was to note at least three things each day. By the time of his next appointment the following week, John was amazed that he had managed to record so many positive things amidst his bleak situation. The sun shone one day warming his skin and calming his mind. Another day, he was phoned by a friend with whom he had not been in contact for a long time. He had had emotional support from his family. He had managed to work half-time that week, which gave him a feeling of being in control of his life. The list was long.

John's attitude slowly changed. He realised that despite everything, there was much good to be enjoyed in his life, even though his condition was serious. The worries were still there, but he had learned to pay less attention to them.

Encouraging thoughts

When worries are oppressive, it can be helpful to find alternative, encouraging thoughts to replace them. Imagine that you are anxious and can't manage to relax. Perhaps you are thinking, 'I'll never be well again.' Such thoughts not only make you more anxious and depressed, but also drain your energy. It's important to replace them with positive, encouraging thoughts that can help you towards your goal.

Some encouraging thoughts

'I may never be fully healthy again, but there is some hope of being better than I am just now. And if that doesn't happen, I will have done my best anyway.'

'If I'm not going to be fully healthy again, at least I shall try to make my days as good as possible!'

'There are many people in my position who manage to have a good life nevertheless.'

'Even though I'm anxious just now, I can do something to calm myself, such as calling a friend to invite him/her to come out for a walk. That has worked before, and it will work again.'

'I'm a strong person and can cope with these feelings; they'll soon settle.'

Many people find that even when worrying thoughts come knocking at the door, they fade away after a while. Can you manage to accept that the worries are there, and then ask yourself what use it is to think about them right now, or indeed to think that way at all?

Gradually, you can learn to leave your worries there without wrestling with them or trying to throw them away.

It can be helpful to find a counsellor who can guide you through mental strategies for handling stress and negative thoughts. Your doctor may be able to refer you, or alternatively there are good self-help courses on the internet.

SHOPPING LIST

Healthy fat
Olive oil, linseed oil, rapeseed oil, organically produced butter.

Protein
Eggs, preferably from free-range hens.

Fish and shellfish
Take your pick; most fish and shellfish are healthy food. Wild-caught fish are better than farmed fish, because of their more varied feeding, and plain fish is better than processed fish products such as fish-balls, fish-fingers or fishcakes. There is a wide choice, including salmon, trout, mackerel, sardines (including canned sardines in olive oil), cod, saithe, etc.; plus prawn, lobster, crab, mussel; cod roe.

Meat
Preferably wild meat (of any type);
Red meat in moderate amounts;
Processed red meat in smaller amounts (mince, sausage, burgers, etc.).

Vegetable protein
Lentils, peas, chickpeas, mung beans.

Carbohydrate
Protein bread;
Wholegrain and multigrain products;

Oatmeal, seeds;
Homemade bread or crispbread (low carbohydrate) with seeds, nuts and kernels.

Vegetables
Free choice at the vegetable shelves, with the exception of potato and sweetcorn which are quickly broken down into large quantities of glucose and raise the blood sugar level. Sweet potatoes are a better option than potatoes. (See list of the top ten most effective vegetables.)

Fruit and berries
Oranges, lemons, mandarins, grapefruit, apricots, pomegranates, blueberries, raspberries, cranberries, blackberries, cherries.

Nuts
Walnuts, hazelnuts, almonds, pecan nuts

Mushrooms
Pleurotus, portobello, shitake, maitake, enoki (These may not be readily available in ordinary shops.)

Soya
Tofu, soya beans, soya beansprouts, soya milk.

Herbs and spices
Turmeric, black pepper, oregano, rosemary, mint, thyme, marjoram, basil, ginger, parsley, cinnamon.

Chocolate
70% chocolate or more (86-90%).

Artificial sweeteners
Stevia, sucralose, tagatesse, cocoa sugar.

Drinks
Water (including carbonated water), organic green tea, dry red

wine (less than 5 grams sugar per litre).

LET'S ALL JOIN THE STRUGGLE!

I still remember the answer the oncologist gave me when I asked, 'What can I do myself to improve my prognosis?'

'There's not very much you can do for yourself, other than to follow the usual advice not to smoke, not to drink a lot of alcohol and to eat a normal, healthy diet.'

He probably was thinking that I should not expend energy on changing my diet, which would just be an added burden for me.

His answer disappointed me. I was very keen to do something useful to help myself, and I had already started looking into several measures that looked promising. I can understand his reasoning, if the premise is that a cancer patient has a limited time to live and he doesn't want to deny the patient what pleasures remain or add to his burdens with strict diet or excess physical activity.

However, I think this approach overlooks the importance to a patient of being able to contribute, to regain a feeling of control and purpose. In my own case, I know that physical exercise and a healthier diet, plus reduction of the stresses of daily life, gave me a quality of life better than I had had before the cancer struck me.

The Berlin Marathon was the first step in my struggle. The idea of running a marathon one year after the operations seemed almost impossible, but I knew that it was important to me to have a big, defined goal to strive and work towards. My joy in achieving this was indescribably great.

Every day since the diagnosis has been a step on the way in this struggle.

Both big and small things done every day have given me a sense of purpose and a good feeling of having achieved something, in contrast to the feelings of fear and helplessness that I had thought would fill my days. I now feel grateful every day that I feel well and that I am living a good life with my family and back at work almost four years after my diagnosis (as of january 2020). The large and small steps I have taken have gradually become routine and are no longer experienced as an effort in my fight against cancer.

EPILOGUE

My legs were aching and sweat was trickling down my back. My red shirt was saturated and the water bag on my back was almost empty, but my smile stretched from ear to ear.

The bells of St. Basil's Cathedral rang as we ran into the Red Square. The road to Moscow had been paved with pains and effort, but also with joy, relief, anticipation and achievement. More than two years had passed since it had been decided that I should try this – if I survived. I had phoned my friend Geir Stian to tell him about my illness. His first response was silence; just like the other times I had told people about my cancer, the news was falling on him like a bomb. His reply came after a few seconds:

'O.K., Øyvind. That's sad to hear, but let's think of this as the autumn you fought against cancer and won!'

Just then, before all my subsequent efforts and their positive results, before I dreamt of running the Berlin Marathon, I really had no will to fight.

However, Geir Stian was confident that everything would go well, and I never forgot what he had said but thought about it more and more as I shook off the first shock and came up to the surface again.

We brushed the dust off a shared dream to run from Paris to Moscow, in the footsteps of the legendary Norwegian runner, Mensen Ernst, in fourteen days. We would need to scale down to a more achievable schedule.

As we ran the last few metres into the Red Square, we

were achieving a goal that I had dreamt of but that I had hardly considered possible two years before. Geir Stian and I had run seven marathons between Paris and Moscow – in thirteen days.

I had recovered from being sick and weak, and I realised that since the apparently unachievable goal had been set I had felt calm and joyful, with a sense of purpose and a feeling of achievement, as I worked to make the dream come true. Well aware that I had not been declared fully cured – as I probably never will be – I believed strongly that everything I had been doing in the past two years – which you have been reading about in this book – was the reason that I had managed so well.

I have been sustained by the various strategies described, which have provided a light in the darkness and an inspiration to live life to the full, despite disease and poor prognoses.

I very much hope that my experiences can inspire you to live life to the full, even in the heat of the battle.

Øyvind Torp,
Moscow, August 2018

Would you help me spread the word?

When I got cancer, someone told me about a book; "Anti-cancer", written by David Servan Schreiber. That book meant the world to me and I felt it saved my life.
If you found this book helpful, please leave a review at Amazon. This way, I can get the message out to more cancer patients like

myself.

Visit amazon.com and leave your review with this link:

https://www.amazon.com/review/create-review?
&asin=1655108565

Thank you so much!

- Øyvind

Further reading

Dr. David Servan Schreiber: 'Anticancer – A new way of life,' Editions Robert Lafont, S.A. Paris (2007).
The book that really inspired me to change my own lifestyle. The author writes about his own journey with cancer and what he learned on the way.

Dr. Raymond Chang: 'Beyond the magic bullet, the anti-cancer cocktail,' Square One Publishers (2012).

Oncologist Raymond Chang explains why you need to combine all potential measures to hit cancer most effectively. He discusses effective dietary factors together with drugs and other treatment.

Jack Westman: 'The Cancer Solution, taking charge of your life with cancer,' Archway Publishing (2015).
A doctor whose wife's illness and death from cancer prompted him to study the available research. Westman discovered untapped possibilities in adjustment of diet. An inspiring book about food and cancer.

Travis Christofferson: 'Tripping over the truth,' Chelsea Green Publishing (2017).
An authoritative book that explains why a ketogenic diet is a good idea for people with cancer and investigates the theory of cancer as a metabolic disease.

Thomas N. Seyfried: 'Cancer as a metabolic disease,' Wiley (2012).
The author, who has been a leading cancer researcher for several decades, presents ground-breaking research on cancer as a metabolic disease. He explains why it is wise to cut down carbohydrate intake and reduce calories. This scientific book may be difficult to read, but it presents convincing research findings.

Nina Teicholz: 'The big fat surprise,' Simon & Schuster paperbacks (2014).
The prominent health journalist thoroughly investigates the misleading advice we have been given to avoid eating fat. Read the studies she describes and be surprised at how wrong we have been.

Zoe Harcombe: Subscribe to the website of the researcher who has critically dissected the messages that saturated fat is harmful. www.zoeharcombe.com

Warren Jefferson: 'The healing power of turmeric,' Healthy Living Publications (2015).

Sidharta Mukerji: 'The emperor of all maladies,' Harper Collins Publishers (2011).
The history of cancer from an experienced Indian oncologist.

Neil D. Barnard et al.: 'The cancer survivor's guide, foods that help you fight back,' Healthy Living Publications (2008, 2017). A handbook having much in common with the book you are already holding, with advice about the most effective foods for people who are surviving cancer.

To my fellow medics

I have never been in any doubt that I should follow the oncologists' advice about my treatment. Cancer specialists have more knowledge and experience in this than I have.

I observe, however, that in consultations with cancer patients, there is very little discussion of motivation towards changes of lifestyle. I think there is an unused potential here; it could help some people by slowing the progress of their illness and others by improving their quality of life after diagnosis. It could encourage most patients by giving them a sense of active participation in their own treatment. I think we need to acknowledge that there is much we don't yet know and that the potential combined effect of lifestyle changes and conventional treatment have not been well studied. Despite the lack of fully documented research, the potential advantages appear much greater than the possible disadvantages.

We should not underestimate patients' need to contribute to their own care and treatment. I think we often forget this, and I admit to having often overlooked it in my work with my own patients.

Notes

1 Inger Kristin Larsen: 'Cancer in Norway 2016,' Kreftregisteret.no.

2 P. Gjersvik: 'Verdens helse: Økt forekomst av barnekreft i Europa,' ('The World's Health: Increased Incidence of Childhood Cancer in Europe') in *Tidsskriftet*, (125) 2005 : 188.

3 Institut National de Veille Sanitaire: 'Estimations nationales: tendances de l'incidence et de la mortalité par cancer en France entre 1978 et 2000' ('National Estimates: Trends in the Incidence of and Mortality from Cancer in France between 1978 and 2000'), Ministere de la Santè, de la famille et des personnes handicapées, 2002.

4 T.L. Roth, F.D. Lubin, A.J. Funk, J.D. Sweatt: 'Lasting Epigenetic Influence of Early-Life Adversity on the *BDNF* gene,' in *Biol. Psychiatry* (65) 2009:760-9.

5 J. Williams, R. Blot, E. Tarone: 'Doll and Peto's Quantitative Estimates of Cancer Risks: Holding Generally True for 35 Years,' in *Journal of the National Cancer Institute*, (107) 2015.

6 Helsedirektoratet: 'Utvikling i norsk kosthold 2017' ('Development in Norwegian Diet 2017'), 12/2017.

7 A. Hjartåkr, H. Langseth, E. Weiderpass: 'Obesity and diabetes epidemics: cancer,' in *Adv Exp Med Biol repercussions*, (630) 2008: 72-93.

8 The sugar comes from fruit that has been pressed. To eat an apple is fine, but it takes many apples to produce a litre of juice and the sugar content will therefore be high. Also, in the pressed juice you won't get the fibre from the fruit that would otherwise hinder the absorption of the fruit sugars.

9 Inger Kristin Larsen: 'Cancer in Norway 2015,' Kreftregisteret.no.

10 Robert McCarrison, the leading British nutritional researcher in India at the beginning of the 1900s was one of the most influential people in nutritional research at that time. He wrote that he was very impressed by the health of some of the folk groups in India: 'The Sikhs and the Hunza people are not plagued by some of the diseases we have in the West – including cancer.' He described the differences in diet between these healthy populations and people further south where there was much more disease.

11 B.A. Kaipparettu: 'Crosstalk from non-cancerous mitochondria can inhibit tumor properties of metastatic cells by suppressing oncogenic pathways,' in https://journals.plos.org/plosone/

article?id=10.1371/journal.pone.0061747; R.L. Elliott: 'Mitochondria organelle transplantation: introduction of normal epithelial mitochondria into human cancer cells inhibits proliferation and increases drug sensitivity,' in *Breast Cancer Research and Treatment*, (136) 2012: 347-354.

12 Thomas N. Seyfried: *Cancer as a metabolic disease*, Wiley (2012).

13 D. Hanahan, R.A. Weinberg: 'The hallmarks of cancer,' in *Cell*, (100) 2000:57-70.

14 Margaret Hanausek, Zbigniew Walaszek, Thomas J. Slaga: 'Detoxifying Cancer Causing Agents to Prevent Cancer,' in *Integrative Cancer Therapies*, (2) 2003: 139-144.

15 Elizabeth T. Thomas, Chris Del Mar, Paul Glasziou, Gordon Wright, Alexandra Barratt and Katy J. Bell: 'Prevalence of incidental breast cancer and precursor lesions in autopsy studies: a systematic review and meta-analysis,' https://www.ncbi.nlm.nih.gov/pmc/articles/PMC5712106/.

16 Xin Xu, Jiangfeng Li, Xiao Wang, Song Wang, Shuai Meng, Yi Zhu, Zhen Liang, Xiangyi Zheng, Liping Xieb: 'Tomato consumption and prostate cancer risk: a systematic review and meta-analysis,' in *Sci Rep*, 2016.

17 William W. Li, Vincent W. Li, Michelle Hutnik and Albert S. Chiou: 'Tumor Angiogenesis as a Target for Dietary Cancer Prevention,' in *Journal of Oncology*, Volume 2012, Article ID 879623.

18 M. Inoue, K. Tajima. M. Mizutani et al.: 'Regular consumption of green tea and the risk of breast cancer recurrence: Follow-up study from the hospital-based epidemiologic research programme at Aichi Cancer Centre (HERPACC)' in *Japan' Cancer Letters*, n. 2 2001: 175-82; N. Kurashi, S. Sasazuki, M. Iwasaki, et al.: 'Green tea consumption and prostate cancer risk in Japanese men: A prospective study,' in *American Journal of Epidemiology*, n. 1 2007: 71-7.

19 James W. Daily: 'Efficacy of Turmeric Extracts and Curcumin for Alleviating the Symptoms of Joint Arthritis: A Systematic Review and Meta-Analysis of Randomised Clinical Trials,' in *Journal Tradit. Complement. Med.*, June 2016: 205-233; A. Amalraj, A. Pius, S. Gopi: 'Biological activities of curcuminoids, other biomolecules from turmeric and their derivatives – A review,' in *J. Med. Food.*, August 2016: 717-729; A.B. Kunnumakkara et al.: 'Curcumin inhibits proliferation, invasion, angiogenesis and metastasis of different cancers through interaction with multiple cell signalling proteins,' in *Cancer Lett.*, (2) 2008: 199-225.

20 D.E. Nelson, D.W. Jarman, J. Rehm: 'Alcohol-attributable cancer deaths and years of potential life lost in the United States,' in *American Journal of Public Health*, (4) 2013: 641-648.

21 N. Kurahashi N: 'Green tea consumption and prostate cancer risk in Japanese men: a prospective study,' in *American journal of Epidemiology*, (167) 2007: 71-77.

22 D. Boivin, M. Blanchette, S. Barrette, A. Moghrabi, R. Béliveau: 'Inhibition of cancer cell proliferation and suppression of TNF-induced activation of NFkappaB by edible berry juice,' in *Anticancer Res.*, (27-2) 2007:937-48.

23 Erica K. Sloan: 'The Sympathetic Nervous System Induces a Metastatic Switch in Primary Breast Cancer,' in *Cancer Research*, (18) 2010: 7042-53; Anil K. Sood: 'Adrenergic modulation of focal adhesion kinase protects human ovarian cancer cells from anoikis,' in *Journal of Clinical Investigation*, (5), 2010: 1515-1523; Chris. C. Wolford: 'Transcription factor ATF_3 links host adaptive response to breast cancer metastasis,' in *Journal of Clinical Investigation*, (7) 2013: 2893-2906.

24 S.K. Lutgendorf, A.K. Sood, B. Anderson: 'Social support, psychological distress and natural killer cell activity in ovarian cancer,' in *Journal of Clinical Oncology*, (28) 2005: 7105-13; R. Glaser: 'Stress-associated immune dysregulation and its importance for human health: a personal history of psychoneuroimmunology,' in *Brain, Behavior and Immunity*, (1) 2005: 3-11.

25 Raymond Chang: *Beyond the magic bullet, the anti-cancer cocktail*, Square One Publishers 2012.

26 B.D. Hopkins, M.D. Goncalves, L.C. Cantley: 'Obesity and Cancer Mechanisms: Cancer Metabolism,' in *Journal of Clinical Oncology*, (35) 2016:4277-4283.

27 Center for Disease Control: 'Trends in incidence of cancers associated with overweight and obesity (2005-2014).

28 R.J. Barnard, J.H. Gonzalez, M.E. Liva, T.H. Ngo: 'Effects of a low fat, high fibre diet and exercise programme and breast cancer risk factors in vivo and tumour cell growth and apoptosis in vitro,' in *Nutr. Cancer*, (1) 2006:28-34.

29 P.S. Leung, W.J. Aronson, T.H. Ngo, L.A. Goulding, R.J. Barnard: 'Exercise alters IGF axis in vivo and increases p53 protein in prostate tumour cells in vitro,' in *Journal of Applied Physiology*, (2) 2004: 450-54; R.J. Barnard, T.H. Ngo, P.S. Leung, W.J. Aronson, L.A. Golding: 'A low fat diet and/or strenuous exercise alters the IGF axis in vivo and reduces prostate tumour cell growth in

vitro,' in *Prostate*, (3), 2003: 201-6.

30 Lewis Cantley, Director of the Cancer Research Institute at Weill Cornell Medicine, is a leading director in this field.

31 N. Keum, D.C. Greenwood, D.H. Lee, R. Kim, D. Aune, W. Ju, F.B. Hu, E.L. Giovannucci: 'Adult weight gain and adiposity-related cancers: a dose-response meta-analysis of prospective observational studies,' in *Natnl. Cancer Inst.*, (2) 2015.

32 P.S. Leung, W.J. Aronson, T.H. Ngo, L.A. Goulding, R.J. Barnard (2004): 450-54

33 S. Brundage, N.N. Kirilcuk, J.C. Lam, D.A. Spain, N. Zautke: 'Insulin increases the release of proinflammatory mediators,' in *Trauma*, (2) 2008: 3676-72.

34   J. Marx: 'Cancer Research: Inflammation and cancer: the link grows stronger,' in *Science*, (5698): 966-968.

35 M. Huang, M. Stolina, S. Sharma, et al. : 'Non small-cell lung cancer cyclooxygenase-2-dependent regulation of cytokine balance in lymphocytes and macrophages: up-regulation of interleukin 10 and down-regulation of interleukin 12 production,' in *Cancer Research*, (6) 1998: 1208-16; A. Mantovani, B. Botazzi, F. Colotta, S. Sozzani, L. Ruco: 'The origin and function of tumour-associated macrophages,' in *Immunology Toady*, (7) 1992: 265-70.

36 Marx (2004): 966-968.

37 A.P. Simopoulos: 'The importance of the ratio of omega-6/omega-3 essential fatty acids,' in *Biomedicine & Pharmacotherapy*, (8) 2002: 365-79.

38 A.C. Carr, S. Maggini: 'Vitamin C and Immune Function,' in *Nutrients*, (11) 2017

39   D. Habu et al.: 'Role of Vitamin K_2 in the development of hepatocarcinoma in women with viral cirrhosis of the liver,' in *JAMA*, (3) 2004: 358-361

40 S. Kakizaki et al.: 'Preventive effects of vitamin K on recurrent disease in patients with hepatocellular carcinoma arising from hepatitis C viral infections,' in *J. Gastroenterol Hepatol* (4) 2007: 518-522.

41 S. Wada: 'Chemoprevention of tocotrienols: the mechanism of antiproliferative effects,' in *Forum Nutr*, (61) 2009: 204-216.

42 S.P. Fortmann, B.U. Burda, C.A. Senger et al.: 'Vitamin and mineral supplements in the primary prevention of cardiovascular disease and cancer: an updated systematic evidence review for the U.S. Preventive Services Taskforce,' in *Annals of Internal Medicine* (12) 2013: 824-834.

43   J. Kruk, U. Czerniak: 'Physical activity and its relation to cancer risk: updating the evidence,' in *Asian Pacific Journal of Cancer Prevention* (7) 2013: 3993-4003;

K.Y. Wolin. Y. Yan, G.A. Colditz, I.M. Lee: 'Physical activity and colon cancer prevention: a meta-analysis,' in *British Journal of Cancer*, (4) 2009: 611-616;

S.C. Moore, I.M. Lee, E. Weiderpass at al.: 'Association of leisure-time physical activity with risk of 26 types of cancer in 1.44 million adults,' in *JAMA Internal Medicine*, (6) 2016: 816-825;

T. Boyle, T. Keegel, F. Bull, J. Heyworth, L. Fritschi: 'Physical activity and risks of proximal and distal colon cancers: a systematic review and meta-analysis,' in *Journal of the National Cancer Institute*, (20) 2012: 1548-1561;

T.E. Robsbahm, B. AAgnes, A. Hjartåker et. al.: 'Body mass index, physical activity and colorectal cancer by anatomical subsites: a systematic review and meta-analysis of cohort studies,' in *European Journal of Cancer Prevention* (6), 2013: 492-505;

K.Y. Wolin, Y. Yan, G.A. Colditz: 'Physical activity and risk of colon adenoma: a meta-analysis,' in *British Journal of Cancer*, (5) 2011: 882-885;

Y. Wu, D. Zhang, S. Kang: 'Physical activity and risk of breast cancer: a meta-analysis of prospective studies,' in *Breast Cancer Research and Treatment*, (3) 2013: 869-882;

B.M. Winzer, D.C. Whiteman, M.M. Reeves, J.D. Paratz: 'Physical activity and cancer prevention: a systematic review of clinical trials,' in *Cancer Causes and Control*, (6) 2011: 811-826.

44   L. Pedersen, M. Idorn, G.H. Olofsson, B. Lauenborg, I. Nookaew, R.H. Hansen, H.H. Johannesen, J.C. Becker, K.S. Pedersen, C. Dethlefsen, J. Nielsen, J. Gehl, B.K. Pedersen, P. Straten, P. Hojman: 'Voluntary Running Suppresses Tumor Growth through epinephrine- and IL-6-Dependent NK Cell Mobilization and Redistribution,' in *Breast Cancer Res Treat.*, (6) 2017: 399-408;

C. Dethlefsen, K.S. Pedersen, P. Hojman: 'Every exercise bout matters: linking systemic exercise responses to breast cancer control.' In *Breast Cancer Res Treat.*, (3) 2017: 399-408.

45   C. Dethlefsen, L.S. Hansen, C. Lillelund, C. Andersen, J. Gehl, J.F. Christensen, B.K. Pedersen, P. Hojman: 'Exercise-Induced Catecholamines Activate the Hippo Tumor Suppressor Pathway to Reduce Risks of Breast Cancer Development,' in *Cancer Res.*, (18) 2017: 4894-4904.

46   Quotation from group leader Pernille Højman from The Centre

for Active Health at the National Hospital in Copenhagen.

47 Øyvind Støren, Jan Helgerud, Mona Sæbø, Eva Maria Støa, Solfrid Bratland-Sanda, Runar J. Unhjem, Jan Hoff, Eivind Wang: 'The Effect of Age on the V'O$_2$max Response to High-Intensity Interval Training,' in *Medicine & Science in Sports and Exercise*, (1) 2017: 78-85.

48 Jørn Heggelund, Marius S. Fimland, Jan Helgerud, Jan Hoff: 'Maximal strength training improves work economy, rate of force development and maximal strength more than conventional strength training,' in *European Journal of Applied Physiology*, (6) 2013: 1565-1573.

49 Anders Hansen: *Bli hjernesterk – tren deg lykkelig og smart*, ('Strengthen your Brain – Train Happily and Wisely'), Cappelen Damm, 2016.

50 G. Mammen, et al.: 'Physical activity and the prevention of depression: a systematic review of prospective studies,' in *J. Prev. Med.*, (5) 2013: 649-657.

51 Yusra Al Dhaheri, Samir Attoub, Kholoud Arafat, Synan AbuQamar, Jean Viallet, Alaaeldin Saleh, Hala Al Agha, Ali Eid, Rabah Iratni: 'Anti-Metastatic and Anti-Tumor Growth Effects of *Origanum majorana* on Highly Metastatic Human Breast Cancer Cells: Inhibition of NF-kappa B Signaling and Reduction of Nitric Oxide Production,' in *PLoS One* (7) 2013.
T. Shimizu, M.P. Torres, S. Chakraborty, J.J. Souchek, S. Rachagani, S. Kaur, M. Macha, A.K. Ganti, R.J. Hauke, S.K. Batra: 'Holy Basil leaf extract decreases tumorigenicity and metastasis of aggressive human pancreatic cancer cells in vitro and in vivo: potential role in therapy,' in *Cancer Lett*, (2) 2013: 270-80;
Jessy Moore, Michael Yousef, Evangelia Tsiani: 'Anticancer Effects of Rosemary (*Rosmarinus officinalis* L.) Extract and Rosemary Extract Polyphenols,' in *Nutrients* (11) 2016: 731; Y. Deng, E. Verron, R. Rohanizadeh: 'Molecular Mechanisms of Anti-*Cancer* metastatic Activity of Curcumin,'; in *Anticancer Res.*, (11) 2016: 5639-5647.

52 D.F. Quail, J.A. Joyce: 'Microenvironmental Regulation of Tumor Progression and Metastasis,' in *Nature medicine*, 2013: 1423-1437;
Stéphanie Gout, Huot. Jacques: 'Role of Cancer Microenvironment in Metastasis: Focus on Colon Cancer,' in *Cancer Microenvironment*, 2008: 69-83.

53 C.L. Chaffer, R.A. Weinberg: 'A perspective on cancer cell metasta-

sis,' in *Science*, 2001: 1559-64.

54 S. Shishodia, B.B. Aggarwal: 'Nuclear factor-kappaB activation: a question of life or death,' in *Journal of Biochemistry and Molecular Biology*, (1) 2002: 28-40.

55 Such as imatinib (Gleevec).

56 I. Paur, T.R. Balstad, M. Kolberg, M.K. Pedersen, L.M. Austenaa, D.R. Jacobs, R. Blomhoff: 'Extract of oregano, coffee, thyme, clove and walnuts inhibits NF-kappaB in monocytes and in transgenic reporter mice,' in *Cancer Prevention Research*, (5) 2010: 653-63.

57 R. Sinha, D.E. Anderson, S.S. McDonald, P.J. Greenwald: 'Cancer risk and diet in India,' in *J Postgrad Med*, (3) 2003: 222-8.

58 Y.E. Deng, E. Verron, R. Rohanizadeh: 'Molecular Mechanisms of Anti-metastatic Activity of Curcumin,' in *Anticancer Res.*, (11) 2016: 55639-5647.

59 N. Seeram, L. Adams, Y. Zhang et al.: 'Blackberry, black raspberry, blueberry, cranberry, red raspberry and strawberry extracts inhibit growth and stimulate apoptosis of human cancer cells in vitro.' In *J Agric Food Chem*, (54) 2006: 9329-39;
Gary David Stoner, Li-Shu Wang, Bruce Cordell Casto: 'Laboratory and clinical studies of cancer chemoprevention by antioxidants in berries,' in *Carcinogenesis*, (9) 2008: 1665-1674;
G.D. Stoner at al.: 'Cancer prevention with freeze-dried berries and berry components,' in *Seminars in cancer biology*, (5) 2007: 403-10.

60 Berit NordsNtrand: *Mat med mer* ('Food with More') Fraiva, 2012.

61 M. Yuneva: 'Finding an "Achilles heel" of cancer: the role of glucose and glutamine metabolism in the survival of transformed cells,' in *Cell Cycle*, (7) 2008: 2083-9.

62 Eugene J. Fine: 'Targeting insulin inhibition as a metabolic therapy in advanced cancer,' in *Nutrition Elsevier*, (Oct. 2012).

63 Inspired by Travis Christofferson: *Tripping over the truth*, Chelsea Green Publishing, 2017.

64 R.W. Owen, R. Haubner, G. Wurtele, E. Hull, B. Spiegelhalder, H. Bartsch: 'Olives and olive oil in cancer prevention,' in *European Journal of Cancer Prevention*, (13) 2004: 319-26; J.M. Martin-Moreno, W.C. Willett, L. Gorgojo, et al.: 'Dietary fat, olive oil intake and breast cancer risk,' in *International Journal of Cancer*, (6) 1994; M. Stoneham, M. Goldacre, V. Seagrott, et al.: 'Olive oil, diet and colorectal cancer; An ecological study and a hypothesis,' in *Journal of Epidemiology & Community Health* (10) 2000: 756-60.

65 N. Khan, et al.: 'Targeting multiple signalling pathways by green

tea polyphenol (-) epigallocathecin-3-gallate,' in *Cancer res*, (5) 2006: 2500-2505.

66 N. Kurahashi, et. al.: 'Green tea consumption and prostate cancer risk in Japanese men: a prospective study, in *American Journal of Epidemiology*, (1) 2007: 167.

67 S.C. Larsson, A. Wolk: 'Tea consumption and ovarian cancer risk in a population based cohort,' in *Arch Intern Med*, (22) 2005: 2683-2686.

68 M. Zhang, et. al.: 'Green tea consumption enhances survival of epithelial ovarian cancer,' in *Int J Cancer*, (3) 2004: 465-469.

69 A.A. Ogunleye, et al.: 'Green tea consumption and breast cancer risk or recurrence; a meta-analysis,' in *Breast Cancer Res Treat*, (2) 2010: 477-484.

70 N. Kurahashi, et al.: 'Green tea consumption and prostate cancer risk in Japanese men: a prospective study,' in *American Journal of Epidemiology*, (1) 2007: 71-77.

71 Researchers at the American National Cancer Institute.

72 B.B. Aggarwal, S. Shishodia, Y. Takada et al.: 'Curcumin suppresses the paclitaxel-induced nuclear factor-kappa B pathway in breast cancer cells and inhibits lung metastasis of human breast cancer in nude mice,' in *Clinical Cancer Research*, (20) 2005: 7490-98.

73 J. Ferlay, F. Bray, P. Piesci, D. Parkin: 'IARC Cancer Epidemiology Database,' in *Globocan*, 2000.

74 D. Boivin, M. Blanchette, S. Barrette, A. Moghrabi, R. Béliveau: 'Inhibition of cancer cell proliferation and suppression of TNF-induced activation of NFkappaB by edible berry juice,' in *Anticancer Res.*, (2) 2007: 937-48.

75 H.K. Rooprai, A. Kandanearatchim, S.L. Maidment, et al.: 'Evaluation of the effect of swainsonine, captor, tangeretin and nobiletin on the biological behaviour of brain tumour cells in vitro,' in *Neuropathology & Applied Neurobiology*, (1) 2001: 29-39.

76 A.J. Pan Tuck: 'Phase II study of pomegranate juice for men with prostate cancer and increasing PSA,' in *American Urological Association Annual Meeting, San Antonio*, 2005.

77 C.M. Cover, S.J. Hsieh, E.J. Cram, et al.: 'Indole-3-carbinol and tamoxifen cooperate to arrest the cell cycle of MCF-7 human breast cancer cells,' in *Cancer Research*, (69) 2009: 1244-51.

78 S.V. Singh et al.: 'Sulforaphane inhibits prostate carcinogenesis and pulmonary metastasis in TRAMP mice in association with increased cytotoxicity of natural killer cells,' in *Cancer Research*,

(69) 2009: 2117-25.

79 K. Canene-Adams, B.L. Lindshield, S. Wang, E.H. Jeffrey, S.K. Clinton, J.W. Erdman jr.: 'Combinations of tomato and broccoli enhance anti-tumor activity in dunning r3327-h prostate adenocarcinomas,' in *Cancer Res.*, (2) 2007: 836-43.

80 J. Li, Q.Q. Mao, et al.: 'Legume intake and risk of prostate cancer: a meta-analysis of prospective cohort studies,' in *Oncotarget.*, 2017.

81 American Institute for Cancer Research.

82 M. Hara, T. Hanaoka, M. Kobayashi, et al.: 'Cruciferous vegetables, mushrooms, and gastrointestinal cancer risks in a multicentre, hospital-based case-control study in Japan,' in *Nutrition Cancer*, (2) 2003: 138-147.

83 Y. Kikuchi, I. Kizawa, K. Oomori, I. Iwano, T. Kita, K. Kato: 'Effects of PSK on interleukin-2 production by peripheral lymphocytes of patients with advanced ovarian carcinoma during chemotherapy,' in *Japanese Journal of Cancer Research*, (1) 1998: 125-30.

84 http://ahcccresearch.com/

85 Satoru Arata, Jun Watanabe, Masako Maeda, Masato Yamamoto, Hideto Matsuhashi, Mamiko Mochizuki, Nobuyuki Kagami, Kazuho Honda, Masahiro Inagaki: 'Continuous intake of the Chaga mushroom (*Inonotus obliquus*) aqueous extract suppresses cancer progression and maintains body temperature in mice,' in *Heliyon.*, (5) 2016.

86 A. Jedinak, D. Sliva: 'Pleurotus ostreatus inhibits proliferation of human breast and colon cancer cells through p53-dependent as well as p53-independent pathway, in *Int J Oncol.*, (6) 2008: 1307-1313;

M. Zhang, et al.: 'Dietary intakes of mushrooms and green tea combine to reduce the risk of breast cancer in Chinese women,' in *International Journal of Cancer*, (15) 2009: 1404-8;

Tongtong Xu, Robert B. Beelman, Joshua D. Lambert: 'The Cancer Preventive Effects of Edible Mushrooms,' in *Anti-Cancer Agents in Medicinal Chemistry*, (10) 2012: 1255-1263;

M.L. Ng, A.T. Yap: 'Inhibition of human colon carcinoma development by lentinan from shiitake mushrooms (*Lentinus edodes*),' in *J Altern Complement Med*, (5) 2002: 581-589.

87 D. Sliva: 'Ganoderma lucidum (Reishi) in cancer treatment,' in *Integr Cancer Ther.*, (4) 2003: 358-64.

88 G. Calviello, et al.: 'Antineoplastic effects of n-3 polyunsaturated fatty acids in combination with drugs and radiotherapy; preventive and therapeutic strategies,' in *Nutr Cancer*, (3) 2009: 287-301.

89 M. P. Rahman: 'The importance of selenium to human health,' in *Lancet*, (336) 2000: 233-41.

90 L. Kiremidjian-Schumacher, H.I. Wishe, M.W. Cohen, G. Stotzky: 'Supplementation with selenium and human immune cell functions. II Effect on cytotoxic lymphocytes and natural killer cells,' in *Biological Trace Element Research*, (1-2) 1994: 115-27.

91 Norsk Helseinformatikk ('Norwegian Health Information'), nhi.no.

92 U.N. Das: 'Tumoricidal and antiogenic actions of gamma-linoleic acid and its derivatives,' in *Curr Pharm Biotechnol*, (6) 2006: 457-466.

93 A. Bakshi, et al.: 'Gamma-linoleic acid therapy of human gliomas,' in *Nutrition*, (4) 2003: 305-309.

94 K. Wolkers, et al.: 'Survival of cancer patients on therapy with coenzyme Q10,' in *Biochem Biophys Res Commun*, (192) 1993: 241-245.

95 Liu Hsiao, Huang Yi-Chia, H. Yin-Tzu, Lin Ping-Ting: 'Coenzyme Q10 and Oxidative Stress: Inflammation Status in Hepatocellular Carcinoma Patients after Surgery,' in *Nutrients.*, (1) 2017: 29.

96 W. Zheng, W.H. Chow, G. Yang, F. Jin, N. Rothman, A. Blair, H.L. Li, W. Wen, B.T. Ji, Q. Li, X.O. Shu, Y.T. Gao: 'The Shanghai Women's Health Study: rationale, study design and baseline characteristics,' in *Am J Epidemiol.*, (11) 2005: 1123-31.

97 Jie Li, Qi-QI Mao: 'Legume intake and risk of prostate cancer: a meta-analysis of prospective cohort studies,' in *Oncotarget.*, (27) 2017: 44776- 44784.

98 Norwegian National Nutritional Advice 2011: 'Dietary advice to promote public health and prevent chronic illnesses,'https://helsedirektoratet.no/Lists/Publikasjoner/Attachments/400/Kostrad-for-a-fremme-folkehelsen-og-forebygge-kroniske-sykdommer-metodologi-og-vitenskapelig-kunnskapsgrunnlag-IS-1881.pdf

99 Richard Beliveau, Denis Gingras: 'Foods to Fight Cancer: Essential Foods to Help Prevent Cancer,' Firefly Books, 2016.

100 The list is based on researcher Richard Beliveau's work on which vegetables can be most effective against cancer.

101 Agnetta Anderze 'N-Carlsson, Ulla Persson Lundholm, Monica Köhn, Elisabeth Westerdahl: 'Medical yoga: Another way of being in the world,' in *International Journal of Qualitative Studies on Health and Well-Being*, 9, 2014; Ulla Persson Lundholm, Monica Köhn, Ing-Liss Bryngelsson, Elisabeth Westerdahl, Agnetta An-

derze 'N-Carlsson: 'Medical Yoga for Patients with Stress-Related Symptoms and Diagnoses in Primary Health Care: A Randomised Controlled Trial,' in *Evidence-Based Complementary and Alternative Medicine*, 2013.

102 Store norske leksikon ('Big Norwegian Dictionary')

103 Per-Einar Binder et al.: 'Mindfulness i psykologisk behandling ("Mindf ulness in Psychological Treatment"), Universitetsforlaget ("University Press), 2014.

Index of key words

Growth inhibition

Human genome project (HGP)

IGF-1 (insulin-like growth factor 1)
Immune system
Indole-3 carbinols (I_3c)
Inflammation
Insulin
Interval training

Ketogenic diet
Ketone bodies
Ketosis

Lactate
Lactic fermentation
Lycopene
Lymphatic system

Metabolic processes
Metabolism
Metastasis
Mindfulness
Mitochondria
Mutation

NF-kappa B
New blood vessel formation (angiogenesis)
NK (natural killer) cells
Noradrenaline

Omega fatty acids
Oncogenes

Phenols
Phthalates
Phytochemicals (chemical compounds produced by plants)
Piperin

Polyphenols
Proanthocyanidins
Procyanidins
Programmed cell death (apoptosis)
PSA (prostate specific antigen)

Reactive oxidants
Resveratrol

Salvesterols
Selenium
Signals for cell division
Somatic mutation theory
Sulforaphane
Synergy

TCGA (The Cancer Genome Atlas)
Terpenes
Tumour suppressor genes

Vitamins

Yoga

Made in the USA
Columbia, SC
08 October 2020